The Truth About Health Care

Critical Issues in Health and Medicine

Edited by Rima D. Apple, University of Wisconsin–Madison,
and Janet Golden, Rutgers University, Camden

Growing criticism of the U.S. health care system is coming from consumers, politicians, the media, activists, and health care professionals. Critical Issues in Health and Medicine is a collection of books that explores these contemporary dilemmas from a variety of perspectives, among them political, legal, historical, sociological, and comparative, and with attention to crucial dimensions such as race, gender, ethnicity, sexuality, and culture.

The Truth About Health Care

Why Reform Is Not Working in America

David Mechanic

Rutgers University Press

New Brunswick, New Jersey, and London

Library of Congress Cataloging-in-Publication Data

Mechanic, David, 1936–

The truth about health care : why reform is not working in America / David Mechanic.

    p. ;   cm. — (Critical issues in health and medicine)

  Includes bibliographical references and index.

  ISBN-13: 978-0-8135-3887-7 (hardcover : alk. paper)

  1. Health care reform. 2. Medical policy.

    [DNLM: 1. Health Care Reform—United States. 2. Delivery of Health Care—United States. 3. Health Policy—United States. 4. Insurance, Health—United States. WA 540 AA1 M4t 2006] I. Title.   II. Rutgers series in critical issues in health and medicine.

  RA395.A3M4184   2006

   362.1'0425—dc22   2005035693

A British Cataloging-in-Publication record for this book is available from the British Library.

Copyright © 2006 by David Mechanic

Manufactured in the United States of America

For Nikko and Ruby

Contents

Preface   ix

Introduction   1

Part I   Our Health Dilemma   17

Chapter 1   Is Reform Possible? The Need for Change
and the Forces Against It   19

Chapter 2   What Is Disease and What Should We Treat?   39

Chapter 3   Saving Lives Individually or in Populations   51

Chapter 4   The Murky Challenge of Mental Health   67

Chapter 5   The Activated Patient and the Doctors' Dilemma   84

Chapter 6   The Neglect of Long-Term Care   100

Part II   The Struggle for Solutions   113

Chapter 7   The Quest for Quality   115

Chapter 8   Setting Fair Limits   130

Chapter 9   Restoring Trust in the Health System   143

Part III   The Fork in the Road   159

Chapter 10   The Challenge of Change   161

Chapter 11   Steps in Our Health Future   179

Notes   189

Index   211

I sometimes joke that if we brought together the country's most talented health care experts and asked them to design a system that gives as little value for money as possible they would have trouble coming up with something better than what we currently have. Of course, the situation we find ourselves in isn't a joke. Through no planned design or evil intent, our health care system has evolved in ways that better serve a myriad of economic, professional, and political interests than those of patients and families, and the larger public. Money has always had a place in the provision of medical care. But "big money" has become dominant, and the forces it has unleashed in the quest for profits have had perverse effects. There are many talented and dedicated people working to provide high-quality health care, but the culture of American medicine and the force of prevailing incentives do not play to their goodness.

Many critics rail against shareholder profit and greed in health care, and there is much to justify their frustration and anger. One can write still another book on abuses and even criminality that occurs in this enormous component of the nation's economy. But railing against selfishness only takes us so far. Most medical activity is motivated and sustained by good intentions, but bad outcomes often flow from arrangements and incentives that guide and shape our efforts. And whatever one may think about big money and corporate influence in medicine, it is here to stay and part of the environment that will define our health care future. So while I can empathize with criticisms of the influence of profit seeking on health care trends, and see value in public awareness of excesses, I don't see such critiques as a useful way to think realistically about redesigning health care.

There is no getting around the reality that having forty-six million people uninsured in the most affluent health system in the richest country in the world is unacceptable and shameful. Also clear but less obvious is that without an infusion of new money, our current financing and organizational arrangements cannot achieve the universal coverage that all other modern nations have. We know the United States scores poorly on most indicators of health and mortality, and many factors, including socioeconomic, racial, ethnic, and geographic inequalities, contribute to these abysmal results. We persistently express our unhappiness with this state of affairs, but most of our

efforts to address these problems occur at the margins of our health care system and not by taking more direct action to ensure that everyone has access to
basic health care. We have many of the necessary program elements in place to
achieve universal access but then invariably retreat from establishing realistic
eligibility levels or sufficient funding for the programs. Facing extraordinary
gaps in coverage and inferior health care outcomes, it is ironic that political
discussion now focuses on cutbacks in Medicare, Medicaid, and other programs that provide some kind of safety net. As I write this today, Congress is
seeking to cut some ten billion dollars from projected Medicaid costs over the
next five years, and considering further reductions. We have good reason to be
concerned about the economic problems of Medicare and Medicaid, and the
financing problems they present, but these pressures make it clear that we must
seek more effective and efficient ways to finance services, deliver care, pre-
serve health, and address disparities.

However difficult, we need to look at health care in America realistically
but with a broad lens. Because of their complexity, we ordinarily address
health problems one at a time, but our incremental fixes create new problems.
This happens at the micro as well as the macro level. Seeking to address the
persistent problems of the uninsured, we devise solutions such as refundable
tax credits that penalize those in states where premium costs are high. Concerned about medical errors and fatigue among medical residents, we seek to
reduce their hours of continuing responsibility, which we can agree is a good
thing, but in the process we bring about discontinuities of care for very sick
patients. Hospitals facing problems in recruitment of nurses and maintaining
nursing staffing levels seek to increase work flexibility by allowing nurses to
work three twelve-hour shifts. This works well for many nurses who prefer
these arrangements, but it too breaks continuity. Increasingly, hospitalists substitute for primary care doctors in managing care of patients when they are in
the hospital, and this contributes to quality of care. But the unplanned consequences of all these arrangements are diminished knowledge of the patient and
situations where there is too little familiarity with patients to detect significant
changes in their health status. Some experts believe that this leads to failures
to rescue very sick patients. Clearly, we can't reverse all these various initiatives that have their own rationales, nor would we want to. But we have to
think in broader system terms and consider carefully how crucial functions
can be well performed given all the contingencies and unavoidable arrangements. This is an issue we will encounter repeatedly where the constructive
approach is not to rail against this or that practice but rather to consider how
to reshape care arrangements so that the system functions better for patients.

This book is different than my earlier ones, which hewed more closely to academic conventions. The broad treatment of topics here merits thousands of references and technical citations, but I have consciously limited the notes to a bare minimum, although I believe I have been true to the best evidence available. I have written hundreds of papers that are better documented on many of the topics discussed, but here I draw more broadly on almost half a century of researching, reading, thinking, and writing about our health care system and others. I believe readers who know my work will still find many of the earlier academic strengths but also hear more clearly my voice as to what should be done.

I am especially grateful to Gerry Grob, Allan Horwitz, Lynn Rogut, and Keith Wailoo, who read earlier drafts and made many valuable suggestions. Thanks also to Susan Reinhard, who reviewed the chapter on long-term care. These colleagues have made many valuable suggestions, and their input has helped make the book more accessible to the general reader. I have also been fortunate over many decades to receive research support from The Robert Wood Johnson Foundation and from the National Institute of Mental Health. As National Director of The Robert Wood Johnson Foundation Investigator Awards in Health Policy Research Program, I have been impressed by the need to bring thoughtful policy work to a broader public, and this has contributed to my motivation to go beyond my usual research and seek a wider audience. I'm also grateful to my outstanding assistant, Peg Polansky, who prepared the manuscript and checked references, and to Guldeniz Yucelen, who helped with library work. And to my wife Katie, the girl of my dreams, who always asks the right questions.

David Mechanic
New Brunswick, New Jersey

The Truth About Health Care

Introduction

Why another book on our health care system? There is no lack of books, articles, and Internet sources telling us about the seemingly uncontrollable growth of health care demands and expenditures, the continuing and growing pressures of health costs on federal and state programs such as Medicare and Medicaid and on family household budgets, and the urgent need for reforms on many dimensions. It is nevertheless difficult to come to agreement on what should be done and through what policies. The core purpose of this book is to explore broadly the influences that make achieving consensus and implementing significant change so very difficult. Above all, health and medicine are parts of a larger culture and shaped by many of the forces that motivate perceptions, beliefs, and behavior more generally. Perhaps not obvious, because we take it for granted, is how American values and culture, reliance on markets, and the decentralized character of health care markets and professional groups and their local cultures prevent steps to achieve a more rational system of health promotion, health care provision, and reasonable cost constraints. Ideological differences and the needs and efforts of powerful interests are everywhere apparent.

To see these various forces play out one need look no further than the Vioxx story and the continuing news about the Cox-2 inhibitors. These medications (of which Vioxx is an example), used for arthritic pain and similar pain indications, were said to be superior to standard nonsteroidal anti-inflammatory drugs such as naproxen (known to many through the popular brand name Aleve) because of fewer gastrointestinal complications. First marketed in May 1999 and promoted strongly to doctors and through direct-to-consumer advertising, Vioxx was withdrawn from the market in September 2004 after more than 100 million U.S. prescriptions for it had been filled.[1] Many millions of these prescriptions were routinely given to patients with low risk of gastrointestinal problems who could have easily taken Aleve, aspirin, or other painkillers. The same study that showed some advantage for avoiding gastric side effects (the Vioxx Gastrointestinal Outcomes Research Study [VIGOR] published in the *New England Journal of Medicine* in November 2000) found that patients receiving Vioxx had four times as many heart attacks as those given naproxen, but this received little attention in the marketing blitz, and it was charged that Merck, the manufacturer of the drug, had purposely tried to mislead doctors.[2] In 2001 Eric Topol and his colleagues reported similar cardiovascular dangers for Vioxx and Celebrex[3] and urged that clinical trials specifically examine the cardiovascular risks and benefits of these drugs, but such studies were never initiated.[4] Merck withdrew Vioxx from the market only in late 2004, following a colon cancer study that inadvertently and unequivocally confirmed the association between Vioxx and increased heart attack and stroke deaths. In the period between 2000 and 2004, thousands of patients died because of marketing hype and lack of attention to indications that the Cox-2 inhibitors could be dangerous to the public's health. In the first Vioxx trial, a Texas jury awarded $250 million dollars in August 2005 to a woman whose husband died after taking the drug. In a second trial in New Jersey in November 2005, a jury found that Vioxx had not caused the heart attack of a postal worker after he had used the drug for a short time. Thousands of lawsuits against Merck remain to be adjudicated.

The story about Vioxx and related drugs will continue to unfold with further study and litigation. But it vividly reveals many of the pressures and interests characteristic of our health system. To the extent these drugs reduced gastrointestinal risk, some patients who have difficulty tolerating other painkillers might benefit, and some patients believed these drugs helped them more than alternatives. Moreover, the individual risk, while real, is small, so persons in pain who had difficulty tolerating other drugs might opt for Vioxx or Celebrex despite the risks. Such uncertainties are common in medical care and are used to justify many interventions. A greater difficulty was that the pharmaceutical companies, seeking to maximize markets and profits, downplayed the risks and sought to market these as preferred "everyday" drugs to doctors and directly to consumers. Almost everyone has heard of Vioxx and Celebrex, and patients commonly requested these drugs, seen in television ads, from their doctors. Doctors' views have also been distorted by the hype and biased marketing to them. Even if doctors fully understood the risks, converting patients' requests takes valuable time and risks alienating patients who demand these drugs.

The controversy concerning these drugs has also made clear the limited jurisdiction of the Food and Drug Administration (FDA) in mandating and monitoring post-marketing studies, distortions in budget priorities associated with dependence on the industry for part of its budget, and conflicts of interest among scientific advisors, many of whom are consultants to the industry. In seeking scientific advice on whether Celebrex should be removed from the market, for example, the FDA included among its advisors many scientists and physicians with what seem to some observers as serious conflicts of interest. While the advisory committee narrowly concluded that Celebrex should remain on the market, the majority of those without ties to the industry voted to have it removed. The overall scientific judgment of the committee may not be scientifically tainted, but the appearances of such bias contribute to still another problem, the erosion of trust in government and in medicine.

Pharmaceuticals receive much of the attention, but there are similar issues about appropriate standards and responsibilities for device manufacturers, physicians who use these devices, and the FDA. Some of these concerns have been brought to broader public attention by the publicized failure of implantable cardioverter-defibrillators (ICDs), and a particular model (the Prizm 2 DR) manufactured by Guidant before April 16, 2002. Following the death of a young college student who was implanted with this device, and a number of other instances of failures of the device, Guidant did not inform physicians or patients of the problem, and although the company modified the device, it quietly continued to sell the devices manufactured before these changes.[5] In July 2005, after much public attention, the FDA recalled the early-manufactured Prizm 2 DRs as well as some other models. Although by 2005 forty-three failures had been identified, the number of failures and deaths probably has been significantly underestimated. Like all other companies faced with these issues, Guidant asserts that it has behaved responsibly and ethically. But its credibility is undermined by the fact that one of its subsidiaries, Endovascular Technologies, which manufactured a stent-graft implanted through a catheter, pleaded guilty to ten felony counts in 2003 for lying to the government and concealing thousands of health problems, including deaths, and had to pay more than ninety-two million dollars in fines. Issues around these complicated technologies are difficult for members of the public to learn about and understand, but they must trust that standards and procedures have been set in place by appropriate government agencies to protect them, an important theme that will recur throughout this book.

Developments in the various health sciences and emergent technologies over the past century, and especially over the past several decades, have increasingly influenced how we view life itself, our perceptions of health and what it means to be healthy, and our expectations for and demands on the health system. Such views encompass a wide span, from approaches to assisting fertility and assessing fetal life prospects to managing death and life supports at the end of life. It involves vigorous debates on the nature of life itself and on the morality of abortion, stem cell research, and therapeutic cloning among others. What emerges is part of a reciprocal process in which producers and marketers of health products and services, and even bioethical ideologies, seek to shape our beliefs, aspirations, and desires, and these then play back via our expectations and demands.

As historians of medicine have repeatedly documented, new knowledge, technologies, and drugs lead to new and refined concepts of disease and ideas about needed interventions.[6] Specialties and subspecialties seeking to take advantage of emerging practice opportunities develop around new techniques and approaches.[7] Pharmaceutical and medical products companies attempt to find new markets for their products and participate in the definition of new diseases that their products could treat. They commonly finance professional conferences and consensus groups seeking to define new preventive and treatment opportunities and approaches to treatment. Increasingly, these new products are oriented not only to illness and reducing alleged future risks of disease and disability but also to bodily and mood enhancement.[8] More and more of what were once seen as social, behavioral, or normative aspects of everyday life, or as normal processes of aging, are now framed in a medical context and viewed as targets for medical interventions. Whether wrinkles, breasts, or buttocks, impotence or social anxieties, or inattention in school, they all have become grist for the medical mill. Economic opportunities for entrepreneurs, whether manufacturers or service providers, encourage and reinforce the impetus toward medicalization.

Some of these new treatments and enhancements remain individual consumer items. As they come to be valued, however, there is increasing pressure to make them part of the medical care package covered by insurance. Until a couple of decades ago medicine was defined by whatever doctors decided was necessary, and insurers generally did not question their decisions. But with the proliferation of expensive new technologies and treatments, and the rising costs of health care and health insurance, payers are trying to exercise more leverage about what treatments are justified and how they are utilized. They increasingly demand justification for expensive treatments and use of high-cost services such as nuclear magnetic resonance (NMR) screening or inpatient care. Since most health insurance is provided through employment or government programs, and patients typically pay directly for only a small part of their care, there is continuing tension between the services patients want and demand and the willingness of payers to subsidize them. These pressures are particularly acute in large government programs like Medicaid but are also characteristic of employer-based insurance and remain important and contentious areas of medical care. When people or their loved ones are sick they want everything possible done, however remotely useful. Nevertheless, it is difficult, indeed probably impossible in the long run, to reconcile these wants with willingness to finance care. This is what some call the allocation or rationing challenge. We have yet to establish an agreed-upon framework for making allocation decisions in a way that is acceptable to all of the interested publics—patients and families, professionals, employers, insurers, and government among others. As I will examine in detail later, the reluctance of the American public and many health professionals to accept limitations on care when ill is a core feature underlying our failures to reach rational solutions to our cost dilemmas.

Talking about rationing in the politics of American medical care remains unacceptable, although we do ration in many ways, typically in ways that are not obvious to the general public. Explicit rationing, where patients and doctors had to seek permission for expensive decisions, as was common in the early years of managed care, infuriated many patients and professionals and contributed to the managed care backlash.[9] Although there are now more controls on allocation of care than in past years, the American system remains very much open to patient and professional demands, which contributes to its enormous costs. These demands often seem defensible because there is uncertainty about the value of many medical interventions and there are many conflicting opinions on what measures are best. Some medical interventions offer small incremental advantages over alternatives, but at great cost. Patients who typically are not paying directly for their care commonly insist on the "best" regardless of cost. Much care is not based on reasonable evidence, and care is often inappropriate and overutilized, but not all involved agree on the particulars.

The Uninsured

Expenditures for services and technologies that many experts believe unnecessary or overused contribute to the high cost of insurance, whether provided through employers, by government, or purchased in the individual market. A significant portion of the population is squeezed out of the market because of these very high costs; about forty-six million people have been uninsured, many more have significant gaps in the continuity of their insurance, and still others have important limitations in their coverage, such as the exclusion of prescription drugs or mental health and substance-abuse care. One analysis for the years 2002–2003 estimated that almost one-third of those under age sixty-five were uninsured for part of the twenty-four-month period, with 65 percent uninsured for six months or more.[10] The uninsured are a heterogeneous group by age, employment status, ethnicity, and geography. Yet a majority of those who are uninsured live in a household with an employed member, typically a spouse or parent. Many jobs either do not offer insurance or provide so little financial coverage that what the employee is required to pay to acquire health insurance for the family, or even him- or herself, is not affordable.

The failure to provide universal health insurance is a long-standing theme in American health policy discussions and an embarrassment for the best-financed health system in the world. No other country comes near to spending as much on health care as we do, but all modern nations have developed systems that provide basic coverage for all their citizens. A study of health spending in the United States compared with Organization for Economic Co-operation and Development (OECD) countries in 2002 found that we spent 53 percent more per capita than Switzerland, the next highest cost country, and 140 percent above median expenditures for all OECD countries.[11] American exceptionalism has motivated endless analytic writings but the number of persons uninsured remains a shameful aberration in a system that Americans like to believe is the best in the world. American national health statistics such as mortality rates are mediocre compared with other industrialized nations. While this is due to many factors, there is little question that limited access to medical care for many and disparities in treatment contribute to these poor results.[12]

The United States, compared to most other developed economies, has a large population dispersed over a vast geographic area and marked by extensive social, ethnic, and racial heterogeneity. It is also an immigrant nation that has a large inflow of people from many countries seeking a better life for themselves and their families, many of whom must struggle with the adversities of limited incomes, poor employment opportunities, language issues, and cultural differences. The country also still suffers from the legacy of slavery, and many black Americans remain poor, continue to face discrimination, and are commonly segregated in ghetto communities with social disorganization and poor infrastructures that exacerbate their problems. America is a place of great opportunities, but it is also a place of large and increasing inequalities and differential access to housing, health, and educational resources.

Influences Affecting Health

Health care is an increasingly important factor in health and longevity and is often lifesaving, but health itself depends much more on the conditions of life and the environmental, social, and behavioral factors that affect developmental processes, living, and work, and the promotive opportunities and social adversities that affect the fate of communities and individuals. The factors affecting health are diverse and complex, ranging from genetic endowments to developmental nurturance; from environmental risks and noxious influences to community enrichment and social capital; from demoralization and poor health behavior to active engagement and health-enhancing endeavors. We now widely recognize that how people live, work, eat, exercise, recreate, and socialize are important influences on their vitality and well-being. Extensive research in these areas makes clear that the pathways are complex and interactive and vary at different developmental stages from infancy to old age. But some of the risks are self-evidently simple and account for much sickness and death; these risks include cigarette smoking, excessive use of drugs, alcohol, and other substances, poor diet, inactivity and excessive weight gain, and much more. These individual behaviors are influenced by the immediate environment, the reigning culture, peer pressures, and advertising inducements. They are also influenced by neighborhood risks and opportunities, such as the availability of healthful foods at reasonable prices, safe places to exercise, noxious pollution, traffic density, and crime and victimization.

We have for decades noted how individual health behavior contributes to health and disease, but the emphasis often has been placed on individuals outside the contexts of the environments that shape their behavior. Socioeconomic status, as reflected in education, income, occupation, and residence, is an important influence shaping individual and group responses. Culture, social support, and individuals' social networks are also central in influencing patterns of behavior, potentially sheltering individuals from adversities and motivating positive and healthful ways of living. The field of population health, which seeks to influence health and disease occurrence by modifying community characteristics that affect many individuals, offers a different understanding of how health and disease are shaped and has advantages over an approach solely focused on individuals. This is important for policy, since we come to better appreciate that even such individual behaviors as smoking, drug use, and exercise are not only products of individual decisions but also are influenced importantly by advertising inducements and cues, access to promotive opportunities, and peer culture and normative restraints. Thus, for example, the prices of cigarettes and alcohol affect whether youngsters take up smoking and drinking, and cultural norms and peer attitudes about smoking affect when and where people can smoke and motivation to start and stop.

Challenges of Chronic Disease

With changes in fertility and mortality, immigration, and disease patterns, the experiences and needs of populations change and the medical system, if it is to perform adequately, must accommodate these changes. As fewer people die of infections and acute conditions in early life, people live longer. When increased longevity combines with declining fertility in modern nations, the population itself ages, unless it substantially replenishes the young through immigration. Modern health care is primarily concerned with chronic disease and disability and the challenge of maintaining vitality and function among people with infirmities that have a long gestation. Although, with the dominance of cardiovascular disease and cancer, chronic disease has become the core of health care over the last half-century, the health system itself and health insurance have been slow to adapt from their episodic acute care orientation, which fits better with many of the diseases of earlier eras. The fall in cardiovascular mortality was the most remarkable health advance in the last half of the twentieth century, but cancer and cardiovascular disease still account for approximately half of all deaths and for much of the intensity and cost of medical care. We have been slow in changing our systems of care to provide the care necessary to best promote functioning and prevent disability among those with chronic disease.

Much research and experience demonstrate that chronic care requires a longitudinal perspective and teamwork if good outcomes are to be achieved. It was once believed that primary care clinicians, working in teams with other professionals, would plan and coordinate effective treatment and rehabilitation efforts, but in reality this is the exception more than the rule. The health system is highly fragmented, everyone feels busy and harassed, and few have acquired the skill set or the motivation to tackle chronic disease and disability in a way that maximizes function. Appropriate reimbursement incentives could help, and various efforts to develop pay for performance programs are aimed in this direction. But good care of chronic disease involves much more than money. It requires doctors, nurses, social workers, and others to organize and implement a treatment and rehabilitation plan on a continuing basis and to coordinate their efforts in a consistent and integrated fashion with clear objectives and careful monitoring.

Much chronic care is now orchestrated not by primary care clinicians but specialists in particular diseases such as cardiologists, oncologists, or pulmonologists. In some instances these doctors working with experienced nurses and others develop excellent disease management approaches, but again there is much fragmentation and much falls through the cracks. Difficulties particularly arise when patients have multiple chronic illnesses and the perspective from any single specialty providers may be too limited to deal effectively with the complications of these comorbidities. Medicine is increasingly specialized and segmented. While such specialization has real value in many instances, the absence of a broader general view of patient need can be a significant deficiency. Many efforts continue to adapt the system to the chronic disease challenge, and some teams do outstanding work, but the system overall is poorly integrated, and too often it is unclear who is in charge or, in fact, if anyone is in charge. Whether a patient receives good care or poor care is still, too often, a matter of chance.

The quality of care available for effective management of serious chronic disease is often spotty, but chronic care remains the bread and butter for doctors and nurses, and they work hard to take good care of patients. Chronic care management becomes increasingly problematic as patients acquire multiple illnesses and disabilities and enter the long-term-care system. Patients in long-term care typically have multiple diseases and disabilities, and deficiencies in carrying out routine activities of daily living. They require not only good medical care and rehabilitation services but also much attention to their social situation and needs. Promoting effective health and functioning in this population requires attention to an array of needs from excellent medical care and medication management to nutrition, physical therapy, social activities, and psychological support. Long-term care is the part of the health system that few policy makers are prepared to address seriously, largely because of worries about potential costs. I will examine these important but often neglected issues in a later chapter.

End of life is particularly problematic for persons dying in nursing homes as well as in other institutional settings. Although sophisticated hospice services and pain-management teams have improved matters a great deal, many people experience terrible deaths because their needs and preferences are neglected or ignored. If they are in the hospital near death they are commonly subjected to invasive medical interventions that they do not want and that often add to the misery of their final days. Even living wills and health care proxies are often ignored as physicians proceed with heroic and often pointless interventions. Such behavior may result because busy house staff either do not acquaint themselves with patients' wishes or follow a medical imperative regardless of patient preference. Few hospitals have systems in place to ensure that staff understand patient and family preferences and respect them. In the case of pain management, staff having certain religious beliefs may believe that prescribed treatment is hastening death and resist and sabotage pain team recommendations. End of life poses difficult issues, and interventions have been designed to address them, but with disappointing results.[13] End of life seems to exacerbate the complexities, lack of adequate system design, inadequate staff coordination, failures to respect patient preferences, and confusion that not uncommonly describe other aspects of hospital care.

The Scope of Medical Error

Problems with end-of-life care are the tip of the iceberg signaling the confusions and errors that take place less obviously in the complex processes of hospital and medical care. Between 50,000 and 100,000 people die each year as a result of hospital and medical error, and hundreds of thousands of others suffer injuries or other untoward events.[14] Hospitals are not particularly safe places to be, and their lack of adequate quality-assurance systems would be an acute embarrassment to most other large industries. In the last few years medical error has received much attention. Many organizations and government agencies have begun to address the issue, although progress has been slow. Some of the problems are quite simple, including illegible orders that lead to the administration of the wrong medication or administering medications to the wrong patient. Computerized prescriber-order-entry systems address the legibility issue and provide a check against contraindicated medications and drug interactions. But these systems have to be carefully designed; they have their own problems and are not failure proof. Many hospitals have now adopted their use, but others resist because of the cost of technology and resistance of physicians and staff to change old habits. Other needs involve systems to provide checks in high-risk situations, protocols to ensure that necessary communication among teams and shifts take place, standardized protocols for various types of mislabeling, and many more. In 2003 the National Quality Forum endorsed thirty practices intended to prevent errors and injuries and make hospitals safer.[15]

Quality of care has become a central concern, not only for the hospital but for all settings and clinicians. As studies have documented the variability in care among geographic areas, the failures in providing obviously effective and necessary services, and the provision of much inappropriate and unnecessary care, there has been growing demand that services be evidence based. There is now much measurement of care and assessment of its appropriateness, many evaluations of patient and public responses, and concern with the outcomes as well as the processes of care. The Medicare program and private insurers are experimenting with pay-for-performance initiatives, and some of the large medical groups are putting in place their own quality-assurance systems. This is a continuing and long-term challenge, and there are many barriers to overcome. Many professional organizations, health organizations, and government agencies are involved actively, and much will depend on their ability to work together successfully and collaborate on a common agenda and in a consistent way. I will have more to say about this later.

The Pharmaceutical Revolution

Another area I will explore is the growth of the importance of pharmaceuticals and their increasing role in health care provision and increasing costs. When Medicare and Medicaid were introduced in 1966, most patients with insurance paid for their drugs out-of-pocket, and drug costs were only a small part of medical expenditures. In the ensuing years many more valuable drugs have been developed for the treatment of such conditions as heart disease, cancer, and mental illness, and drug utilization costs have skyrocketed. Now the idea of health insurance without drug coverage seems antiquated, yet many people still lack drug coverage. Medicare did not include coverage of drugs, except when administered directly such as by injection or infusion by health personnel, and as the decades progressed it was apparent that the absence of drug coverage was a significant deficiency of the program. Many were not taking needed drugs because of the financial hardship involved.

A prescription drug benefit has been added to the Medicare program as of 2006. This very expensive addition to the program has been a matter of great controversy and continuing agitation. The benefit brings an important expansion of benefits for many elders but includes significant compromises and concessions to private interests. Especially controversial is the gap in benefit coverage, often described as the "doughnut hole," which leaves those with high, but not the highest, drug costs without significant protection. This is irrational as health policy, but the motivation was to keep total expenditures for the benefit in check. Other provisions of the legislation increased the costs of the program by providing large subsidies to private health plans to offer prescription coverage and to employers to retain coverage already being provided to retirees. This seemed necessary to policy makers to make the plan work as a privately administered program, a strong commitment of the Bush administration. Although the program is advantageous to enrollees with very low incomes, some joint Medicare and Medicaid enrollees whose coverage under the legislation will shift from Medicaid to Medicare may fare less well under the new legislation in some states. Many elderly find the program confusing.

A highly controversial aspect of the legislation was the prohibition on Medicare to use its great financial leverage to negotiate drug prices, an approach used by large governmental purchasers in most countries and by the Veterans Administration and state Medicaid programs in the United States. Many saw this as an inappropriate payoff to powerful pharmaceutical interests, while others justified it as a protection of pharmaceutical research and development. The new Medicare pharmaceutical benefit, like much else, illustrates the importance of culture, ideology, politics, and special interests in the making of health policy.

An Uncertain Future

As I write this, America has been engaged in a major debate on the future of our Social Security program. This is more than a bit ironic since Social Security is financially secure for decades ahead and much less of an impending problem than Medicare and Medicaid, whose costs are accelerating rapidly and putting great pressures on federal and state budgets. Moreover, as we will explore throughout this book, our decentralized and open-ended health care system, continuing innovations in knowledge and technology, the aging of the population, the entrepreneurialism of the market, and the expansion of consumer demand as the media advertise promising new possibilities will put great upward pressures on health care costs. In coming decades the growth of medical care costs will exceed overall economic growth and be a source of financial and political problems.

As we progress into the twenty-first century we face many opportunities, uncertainties, and threats. No one can foresee how forces will interact or how global environmental, economic, technological, and political factors will play out. We are increasingly part of a global community, and events, however far away, can very rapidly affect situations here. Diseases travel rapidly around the globe and can devastate large areas and populations. AIDS, although under some control here so that we now think of it as a chronic disease, continues to devastate many populations around the world. As we learned in the Severe Acute Respiratory Syndrome (SARS) outbreak, the occurrence of a life-threatening disease in China, Vietnam, or anywhere else can spread rapidly around the world. Future influenza pandemics are inevitable and it is estimated that if the H5N1 (the so-called bird virus) should become the next pandemic strain as many as 1.7 million people would die in the United States and 180 million to 360 million people would die globally.[16] The World Health Organization has urged increased preparedness, noting that this virus poses a continuing and potentially growing threat.[17] Scientists have been working to develop a vaccine and have promising results, but many problems continue. These present and future threats make international cooperation increasingly essential and require not only vigilance but also thoughtful health actions that do not exacerbate problems. For example, the promiscuous use of antibiotics, for medical care in instances where they have little value and in animal feed that eventually enters our food stream, increasingly allows disease agents to develop resistant strains and reduces our effective instruments to combat disease. There is evidence of alarming increases in hospital infections resistant to antibiotics, estimated to be as high as 50 to 60 percent of the more than two million such infections each year in U.S. hospitals.[18]

Health care policy, as well as health policy more generally, must be thought about broadly in terms of determinants and interventions. Both in promoting health and treating disease we must give attention to the many factors that play a part, including war, poverty, environment, exploitation, and denial of female education and opportunities for empowerment. The quality and safety of the food supply and potable water are central to healthy eating, adequate nutrition, and life itself; a clean and safe environment facilitates community participation and exercise and protection against injury and disease; the incentives and constraints in communities, embodied in norms and social policies, affect use of substances, positive health behaviors, and safe sexual behavior. Health is extremely complicated, and to understand it we study it in smaller pieces. But we also have to understand how to bring the pieces together so that policies move toward common goals and in consistent directions. Health is, of course, not the only priority or even the most important one in all circumstances. But without health our opportunities to pursue and enjoy other aspirations are diminished and even impossible.

Like much else in American politics, health care discussion has become very much polarized, and the public has less a sense of whom to trust than in past times. The public is bombarded with conflicting images and information, eminent doctors disagreeing on many issues of treatment and policy, descriptions of high-profile medical lawsuits, and much advertising promoting the virtues of drugs and treatments. We will never go back to the time when the medical profession spoke with one voice, nor should we want to, but we should aspire to having a framework that inspires more trust and public legitimacy. There is little doubt that however much the public values medical progress it often has difficulty distinguishing between real advances and hype. The medical profession itself has become fragmented, and its leadership has much eroded. Developing a new medical professionalism fitted to a very different environment than in the past and forging a more collaborative relationship with other health professions remain big and challenging tasks for American medicine. Efforts are now in process, early in their gestation, and they will need much support and nurturance.

The chapters that follow focus on various challenges in this very large, complex, and expensive enterprise that some describe as a system and others as a nonsystem. There are hundreds of important issues, some largely ideological, others very technical. In choosing among these issues I focus more on some that have received less attention in general discussions of health care such as population health, trust, rationing, long-term care, mental health, and the changing roles of doctors and patients. I focus less on the details of such important issues as insurance coverage, financing of health care, or controversies about restructuring such important national programs as Medicare and Medicaid because they are already receiving a great deal of discussion. I wish to achieve a broadening of our understanding of health policy issues and challenges and how to address them more constructively.

As we move among themes, the role of varying interests remain central. Discussing special interests evokes in many peoples' minds nefarious influences with undue power who use their political networks, campaign contributions, and financial clout to gain decisions advantageous to them and exploitive of others. Certainly, there are many powerful interests in medicine, from health insurance plans and health science centers to pharmaceutical firms and other big businesses, and they use their money and influence to try to shape health care to their advantage. But in a broader sense, the clash of interests in politics and the marketplace define the American way and its pluralistic orientations, with myriad groups seeking to influence public policy. Decision making can be seen, thus, as something like a tug-of-war, with various groups building coalitions and alliances that they believe will further their objectives. These objectives are often money and profits achieved by a variety of means ranging from selling more products and services to getting higher reimbursements and income, but they extend well beyond this to such concerns as improving quality of care, expanding research and providing services for persons with many specific diseases, building a stronger safety net for the poor, enhancing the status and work conditions of particular professions, reducing regulation of businesses, and much more. Organizations engaged in health care politics include not only Blue Cross, Anthem, Aetna, and United Healthcare but also the AFL-CIO, the Kaiser Foundation Health Plan, and the Chamber of Commerce; not only the American Medical Association, the American Hospital Association, and the American Nursing Association but also specialty groups and more specialized hospital and nursing organizations; not only the American Cancer Society, the American Public Health Association, and the National Alliance for the Mentally Ill but also AARP and Families USA. There are thousands of organized associations, local organizations, political action committees (PACS), consumer groups, and churches, among others, who have a hand in health politics and policy.

A unifying theme is the crucial roles that culture, ideologies, values, and interests have in shaping how dilemmas are conceptualized and how these frames encourage or inhibit consideration of particular kinds of remedies. Our tendency to see solutions in individualized rather than in communal forms contributes to our failures to make sufficient progress in implementing rational systems to provide health insurance for all, to reduce hospital and medical error, to manage chronic disease and long-term care appropriately, to implement practices based on good evidence and not just wishful thinking, and to allocate care in equitable and effective ways. How we frame our challenges affects our ability to evaluate and introduce needed new technologies and innovations such as improved information systems and computerized patient records, and our capacity to control rising costs due to use of untested and ineffective interventions. Culture, ideologies, and interests will always shape the context and make some irrationalities inevitable, but thoughtful solutions that bring interests together offer opportunities for progress on many fronts. Only a fool believes that it is possible to foresee all that lies ahead or that anyone has all the answers. It is inevitable that we will have to muddle through to a considerable extent. It is to be hoped that we can do so more rather than less elegantly.

Part I

Our Health Dilemma

The first section of this book examines the many sides of our health dilemma. The chapters that follow explore varying facets of our future health care challenges and how myriad interests influence the definitions of health and disease, approaches to prevention and treatment, and the financing and organization of health care itself. Many of the problems we face, such as high rates of uninsured persons, the uncontrolled expansion of new and untested technologies, the erosion of primary health care, and the neglect of mental health and long-term care, are in many ways products of how we as a nation organize ourselves economically and politically and how the marketplace unleashes entrepreneurial activities of every kind. It explains why we have such innovative energy but end up paying so much for interventions of little value. It also helps explain why such phenomena as alternative and complementary medicine can prosper alongside robust growth of the traditional medical sector.

Despite its size and sophistication, American medicine is built around local markets and culture, and a highly individualized perspective. The public thinks in terms of personal stories and anecdotes and not in terms of populations and statistics. We go to great lengths to save individual lives at enormous cost and with great compassion, but we care much less about policy initiatives that save many more anonymous lives and at much lower cost. This is the dilemma of population health and how we can structure our health investments to promote health and well-being in populations, prevent illness, and enhance function and physical vitality. It also relates to social disparities of all kinds, from class and race to geography and gender, and how health initiatives might contribute to a more equal society.

The advances in science and technology that inform medical care and public health and shape new public demands, and associated costs, increasingly confront an incompatibility between how medical care has been traditionally organized in the United States and new medical possibilities. We want to bring to patients new interventions of value but prevent abuse, waste, and injuries. We want practice to reflect what is known to be effective, not what physicians are simply in the habit of doing. We want to deliver the safest and most effective drugs, not simply provide those that are effectively marketed and have wide name recognition. We want to have patients as informed partners in care but avoid having advertising hype determine the treatments they receive. This requires new ways of organizing doctors and other health professionals, and skillfully using information technologies to inform and facilitate patient care. Providing an understanding of these challenges is the task for the first six chapters of this book.

Chapter 1

Is Reform Possible?

The Need for Change and the Forces Against It

Having experienced serious back pain for more than forty years, despite back surgery some twenty-five years ago, I follow the back pain literature with much personal interest. In the 1980s I cochaired an Institute of Medicine (IOM) committee on pain, disability, and chronic illness and had an opportunity to work with many experts in the area and to study the literature. In our IOM report we noted the lack of strong evidence for back surgery in most instances of back pain and in the absence of a major neurological deficit.[1] We did note that while surgery often helps persons with acute sciatica resulting from a herniated lumbar disc, surgery often was unnecessary in the absence of neurological deficit, and longer-term outcomes of surgery for sciatica were no better than from medical treatments. We found even less support for surgical treatment of low back pain in many other instances or for repeated back surgeries.

Back pain is one of the most common medical complaints and over the years complex surgical interventions for back problems have increased dramatically. Spinal-fusion surgery, for example, rose by 77 percent between 1996 and 2001, probably as a result of population changes, technological advances, uncertainties concerning criteria for intervention, and financial advantages for surgeons, hospitals, and manufacturers of medical devices.[2] Spinal-fusion surgery is a multibillion-dollar business and more expensive than simple laminectomy. Aware that spinal-fusion surgery was often unnecessary, overused, and had more complications than other back surgery, the federal Agency for Health Care Policy and Research (now renamed the Agency for Healthcare Research and Quality) sought to bring evidence-based rationality to this area, enlisting a multidisciplinary panel to exhaustively view the best studies and develop

guidelines for managing acute back problems. For most instances and indications the panel recommended nonsurgical approaches.

The guidelines did not please some orthopedic surgeons, for whom back
surgery is bread and butter. Although the American Academy of Orthopaedic
Surgeons® endorsed the findings, the North American Spine Society inspired
a letter-writing campaign to members of Congress charging the research team
with bias and ineptitude.[3] This was followed by organization of a lobbying
organization, named the Center for Patient Advocacy, that sought to eliminate
funding for the federal agency, which in the view of most observers familiar
with its work was doing an admirable job of developing credible practice
guidelines. Following this lobbying, the House of Representatives eliminated
funding for the agency in its 1996 budget. After much effort by advocates, the
Senate reinstated funding, although the final budget cuts for the agency were
substantial. The agency, which had as its mandate research on medical care
outcomes, ended its guideline work concluding that it was more properly a
task for others. Similarly, the Congressional Office of Technology Assessment,
established in 1972 to advise Congress on science and technology issues
including important health care technologies, irritated private-sector interests
and was eliminated at about the same time.[4] The issue we face is how to build
a rational and unified health system when the public interest so easily yields
to private interests who have their own axes to grind and oppose independent
objective assessment.

Critics of health care in the United States often refer to it as a nonsystem.
They commonly point to the fact that we spend far more per person than any
other country in the world, have some forty-six million people uninsured, have
mediocre health outcomes as reflected by our infant and adult mortality rates,
experience large race and social disparities, have much fragmentation in care
processes, do poorly in both preventive efforts and efforts to promote good
health, and get much less value for money than we should. Supporters of
American health care in contrast point to the high quality of our research and
medical education efforts, the talented people we attract and train for health
care work, the impressive infrastructures of hospitals and other health care
institutions, our high levels of technological innovation, and the wide range of
choices we offer, at least to those who are well insured or who can afford care.
The challenge is whether we can use our rich resources, inventiveness, and
many other assets to develop a system that better serves the entire population
and that produces higher-quality care and better outcomes. Is it possible to
bring many of the components that individually have many merits into a well-
functioning overall system?

Basic to this challenge is the understanding that delivering high-quality care depends on well-designed systems as well as competent, well-trained, and motivated people. Many patients and professionals continue to view medical care as consisting of relatively simple relationships between clinicians and patients, depending primarily on the knowledge, skills, and professionalism of the clinician. It is not difficult to understand why doctors see themselves as at the center of care, but any complex treatment depends on a wide range of people in supporting roles, and coordination and teamwork among many participants. Success at the bedside depends on systems being in place for communication, coordination, monitoring, following-up, and keeping many threads together.

Errors are made in many ways, from the most mundane, such as nurses unable to read the physician's illegible instructions, to the most shocking, as when the wrong patient is subjected to dangerous surgical and other procedures. Mark Chassin and Elise Becher very thoughtfully have analyzed one such instance in which a sixty-seven-year-old woman mistakenly underwent an invasive cardiac electrophysiology study after having been admitted to a teaching hospital for a cerebral angiography. About an hour into the invasive intervention it became clear that this was the wrong patient. In meticulously analyzing this error, the analysts identified seventeen distinct errors, but no single one could itself have caused the event. Writing for their medical colleagues, they note, "The most important latent conditions in this case include failures of communication, teamwork and identity verification. Perhaps the most striking feature of this case—one that will be familiar to all clinicians who have worked in large hospitals—is the frighteningly poor communication it exemplifies. Physicians failed to communicate with nurses, attendings failed to communicate with residents and fellows, staff from one unit failed to communicate with those from others, and no one listened carefully to the patient."[5]

Success at the population level also requires a systematic view of care arrangements and ways of ensuring access, follow-up, and continuity, clear definitions of responsibilities and accountability, and preparation for a wide range of contingencies. Insuring community health requires a broad understanding of risks and a coherent public health structure for prevention, health promotion, and controlling disease spread. Overcoming an individual focus and understanding how teamwork and established processes increase opportunities to achieve aspirations and perform better are basic to all complex industries. These ideas are well understood in many specialized endeavors common to complex medical and surgical care, as, for example, in transplantation services or burn units, but such thinking is not very prevalent in more commonplace medical settings or, even more importantly, in how we organize our health services overall.

The Cultural Context of Care

The stalemate in achieving broader health reform is conditioned by two competing worldviews that are difficult to reconcile and are increasingly polarizing. There are those, mostly identified with the Republican Party, who view health care as fundamentally no different from other products and services and whose provision they believe is best optimized through a competitive marketplace with minimal regulation. Many are sincerely concerned with the problems of persons with limited income and no health insurance and support programs to alleviate these problems, but they do not view health care as a "right." They generally favor strong emphasis on individual responsibility, fee-for-service medicine, and cost sharing as a means of encouraging prudent decision making in the use of health care services. The contrasting view, more identified with the Democratic Party, sees health care as different from most other goods and services, as a public obligation and individual right, and a form of service that does not prosper in an unregulated marketplace or with strong profit-making incentives. This group favors national health insurance, and many favor a single payer, as in Medicare and Health Canada, health care approaches with government playing a significant role in financing and regulating health care. Given the relatively equal balance of political influence in the country and in Congress, these ideological differences create an unbridgeable divide that stalls and sidetracks efforts at overall reform.

The values and ideologies of individuals also strongly influence how health issues play out. Americans tend to be individualistic, distrust government, and believe competitive markets to be more innovative and efficient than any planning models. While they have differing views on the role of government in health care, they feel strongly about choice and their presumed right not to be limited in choice, especially in their choice of physicians.[6] Many who receive their insurance through their employers have no choice of plan, particularly those who work in small firms, but the preference for choice is, nevertheless, strong, and studies repeatedly find that patients who select their plans and clinicians report more satisfaction with them than those who do not have those choices. Americans also feel strongly about taking action and attacking problems and are not inclined toward "watchful waiting" and "fatalism." We have a "can do" culture, and Americans facing illness in themselves or their loved ones want to try anything that offers hope, however unproven or however expensive.

Underlying many of our problems is the persistent and growing problem of the uninsured.[7] In addition to the almost 46 million consistently without insurance in 2003–2004, an additional 37 million people lacked insurance for at least part of the time. Many others are significantly underinsured, with high cost sharing, significant limitations on benefits, and often a lack of coverage for basic services such as prescription drugs, medical appliances, mental health, substance abuse services, and rehabilitation. The uninsured are not entirely without care or dying in the streets, as foreign observers sometimes believe, but they receive significantly less care than insured people, often receive care late and in more expensive locations such as emergency rooms, and when they receive care it is on average less intensive and of lower quality. Thus it is not surprising that the uninsured suffer persistence of their illnesses, disability, and increased mortality.[8] A Commonwealth Fund survey estimated that an additional 16 million persons between the ages of nineteen and sixty-four were underinsured in 2003 as measured by medical expenses that put a strain on living expenses. Such persons resembled the uninsured population in restricting their use of medical services and were much more likely to forego needed medical care than those with better coverage. More than one-third reported having to change their way of life to pay medical bills, and almost half had to deal with collection agencies concerning unpaid medical bills.[9]

Increasing Demands, Costs, and Entrepreneurial Activity

The broader context in which health care reform must be addressed is a difficult one. Health care is now approximately 16 percent of gross national product (GNP), and more than half of all expenditures come directly from large government programs such as Medicare or Medicaid and insurance coverage of public employees, and indirectly from large tax subsidies to employers and employees. The projected growth in federal spending due to changes in medical knowledge and technology, the aging of the population, entry of larger proportions of the population into health entitlement programs, and new pharmaceutical benefits under Medicare faces push-backs because of the large and growing federal deficit and strong resistance to increased taxes. The $1.9 trillion health industry, projected by actuaries at the Centers for Medicare and Medicaid Services to grow to more than $3 trillion by 2012,[10] provides a livelihood for a significant part of the population and large corporate and professional interests, so there is much resistance to changes that would reduce anyone's share. Many of the cutbacks in employer and governmental health commitments have resulted in shifting more costs to patients and reducing payments to health care providers. Both of these approaches face continuing resistance and aggressive lobbying.

At the same time, momentum in knowledge and technology forges ahead, promising abundant new possibilities to extend life, improve function, and enhance personal performance.[11] Advances in genetics, nanotechnology, information sciences, biomaterials, and many other areas feed the health aspirations of the public. Thousands of companies seek to capture a share of health spending by developing new technologies and products, encouraging new needs and demands, and marketing their products aggressively. The emergence of a more competitive marketplace in health, in what continues as a relatively open-ended expenditure environment, encourages consumer interest in a dazzling range of new services, including full-body screening to detect disease, parts replacements, and numerous ways to enhance attractiveness, vitality, and youthfulness. The definitions of health and disease are themselves arbitrary, and the development of new products, whether drugs or other treatments, encourages the definition of new diseases. The increasing medicalization of what were once regarded as normal processes of aging and common problems of living makes all but physical vigor and comfortable adjustment seem a bit pathological. There is, of course, much of value embodied in these developments and trends, but we lack clear and agreed-upon ways of separating what is useful from what is wasteful and even harmful. Science helps us to establish what is effective, but there is much uncertainty, values about desirable end-states vary, and the relevant sciences have yet to fully achieve legitimacy among many who believe the market and individual choice should reign. With the abundance of information outlets in a free society, consumers hear many voices influencing their preferences and demands.

The Momentum of Technology and Its Imperatives

The public greatly values and supports new medical knowledge and technologies, but premature promotion, prior to adequate assessment, exposes persons to costly interventions and diagnoses of diseases they may not really have and treatments that may harm them.[12] Improved imaging technologies have been a remarkable advance in recent decades, and computerized axial tomography (CAT), magnetic resonance imaging (MRI), and positron emission tomography (PET) scanning are increasingly prevalent not only for diagnostic assessment but also for preventive screening purposes. Increasingly, physicians identify bodily indications that are not well understood but lead to definitions of diseases that may not really exist, and interventions that have not been determined to be useful. The technological imperative encourages treatments that may be wasteful and even harmful. Evidence from a range of studies indicates that too much medical care, just like too little, can be harmful.[13] But we have no agreed-upon "sheriff" to establish legitimate criteria for too little or too much, and much uncertainty remains as to what is and is not worth doing.

There are numerous examples of instances where searching for and treating indications from refined testing when the patient has no symptoms leads to treatments that offer no known value and can cause harm. Elliott Fisher and H. Gilbert Welch describe some of the instances where such testing lead to pseudodisease and harm by labeling.[14] They define pseudodisease as conditions "that would never become apparent to patients during their lifetime without the diagnostic test." This idea is not new. In a classic paper written nearly four decades ago, Abraham Bergman and Stanley Stamm reported how mothers responded to reports that their children had heart anomalies, which had no medical significance, by treating them as if they were ill and restricting normal activities.[15] As Fisher and Welch note, "It is increasingly clear that the population with an occult disease is many times larger than the population destined to become sick from it. Microscopic examination of specimens from individuals without known cancer nonetheless reveals a high prevalence of the disease: a third of adults have pathologic evidence of papillary carcinoma of the thyroid, as many as 40% of women in their 40s may have ductal carcinoma in situ of the breast, half of men in their 60s have adenocarcinoma of the prostate."[16] As Richard Deyo and Donald Patrick describe, surgery is needlessly extensive and commonly ineffective.[17] Among the many examples they note of unsuccessful surgical intervention are radical mastectomy for breast cancer, internal mammary artery ligation to increase blood supply to the heart, arthroscopic surgery for arthritis of the knee, episiotomy during childbirth, and fetal-cell therapy for Parkinson's disease. Tonsillectomy is a classic example.

The organization and financing of medical work and the ways we implement medical innovation exaggerate these problems. Pharmaceutical companies make profits by marketing new drugs; professionals increase incomes by promoting new conditions and treatments; specialties, new subspecialties, and specialty clinics and hospitals proliferate around highly profitable interventions; clinicians, most still paid on a fee-for-service basis, earn more by performing more services and particularly those technical ones that bring larger reimbursement. Entrepreneurs, manufacturers, and marketers of medical devices and supplies increase their profits by promoting new, more expensive products, often no better than existing, less costly ones. Increasingly, drugs and treatments are promoted by aggressive direct marketing to consumers through the media and the Internet. Many participants, each motivated by their own interests, work toward increasing the scope of new demands and contribute to aggregate expenditures for care. Some of what is promoted is valuable and even lifesaving; some of it is worthless and even harmful. But it all works to push costs up. Government and health plans attempt to push back, but special interests and public pressure to cover new treatments can be difficult to resist.

From the patient side, the emergence of new screening and preventive technologies that are marketed pose psychological issues. People cherish their health and have been urged to identify risks early so as to prevent more serious problems later. Thus, they are receptive to screening technologies such as body imaging, prostate-specific antigen (PSA) testing, CT lung cancer screening, and the like. Medical entrepreneurs market these technologies, often well before there is evidence of their value or indication that they truly promote health. Screening takes patients on an inevitable trajectory. Once patients are told they might have a serious disease such as cancer they find it difficult to resist the next step on the diagnostic and treatment trajectory, although the costs and dangers might exceed any likely benefits. This is particularly characteristic of American patients, who have been encouraged to be active agents.

There is uncertainty about the value of much of prevalent screening, and strong differences of opinion. The science, also, is typically not definitive, but entrepreneurs and physicians act aggressively on results from small and often poorly designed studies, particularly when economic opportunities are apparent. The history of hormone replacement therapy (HRT) should provide a cautionary tale. Millions of women were receiving HRT for years, encouraged by intense pharmaceutical promotion before more definitive and better-designed randomized trials contradicted suggestions from small clinical studies and indicated that the preventive treatment probably did more harm than good. The story of PSA testing for prostate cancer is increasingly murky, and there is still no persuasive evidence that the intrusive interventions that are commonly pursued, and that pose serious dangers to quality of life, actually save lives. Yet many men are convinced that PSA testing saved their lives, and urologists, who build their livelihood on such procedures, do little to dissuade them. Even the value of mammography, for which there is more persuasive evidence, has been questioned in careful meta-analyses, systematic reviews of research trials, done in Europe and published in the prestigious medical journal the *Lancet*.[18] In all the instances noted there have been at least defensible reasons for pursuing preventive efforts, but in other instances imaging is used in "search and destroy" missions encouraged more by economic motivations than by any serious evidence.

Aborted Efforts at Reform

A perennial area of analysis among scholars is the failure of the United States
to enact a system of universal health insurance, an arrangement present in all
other developed nations. The lack of a well-organized system transcends the
basic problem of insurance coverage. Even those fortunate enough to have
superior coverage can suffer from a highly fragmented and uneven pattern of
services that invites medical and hospital errors that complicate many illnesses and result in many preventable deaths and injuries.[19]

Our health care arrangements are often unfriendly to both patients and
professionals. Patients with complex problems often find it baffling to navigate
the services available with its poorly coordinated outpatient departments, clinics, ambulatory facilities, specialists, primary care doctors, and a range of supportive and complementary practitioners. When seriously ill, they often find
communication and coordination among clinicians involved in their care poor
and have difficulty identifying who is responsible for their care and who can
integrate the efforts of various caregivers. Communication is poor not primarily
because clinicians don't care but more because of system failures that lead to
breakdowns in planning and coordination. Similarly, clinicians feel besieged
by competing demands, conflicting objectives, incentives that discourage quality, and excessive regulation. They commonly view their autonomy and professional integrity as being under attack, and many increasingly feel their
incomes threatened as well.

Many efforts were made over the past century to introduce more organized national health care programs.[20] After the more recent failure of the
Clinton health care plan in the early 1990s, employers and state governments, faced with increasing health care costs, turned to managed care organizations and care management strategies to contain the growth of medical
care costs. During the early years of managed care, the strategies used were
somewhat rigorous, often restricting choice of physicians and sites of care,
requiring primary physician "gatekeeping," reviewing utilization of specialty
referral, and instituting prior authorization for expensive tests and treatments. Health care plans as they moved into managed care were also tough
on physician groups and hospitals, bargaining hard on reimbursement
arrangements and driving down prices. There was much badmouthing of
health maintenance organizations (HMOs) and managed care by professionals who saw their incomes and autonomy at risk and by patient advocates
who were concerned about limits on choice and use of services. The backlash
against managed care is now history, and while we may not have seen the end
of managed care, as some have argued, we certainly see it watered down to

"managed care lite."[21] We have also seen an upturn in costs of care and insurance premiums.

The managed care backlash tells us a great deal about American health care and the difficulties of reforming it. The research literature on health care delivery in general, and HMOs and managed care in particular, show great variability in performance within both HMOs and fee-for-service traditional practice. In the aggregate, HMOs and managed care offer some advantages in terms of lower cost, less paperwork, and more preventive medicine, and some disadvantages, such as less choice and flexibility. But on the whole, the differences in preventive care, access, satisfaction, and quality within each model of care are greater than comparative outcomes across models. The differences in quality between HMOs and traditional fee-for-service medicine can be said to be pretty much a wash.[22] Thus, performance alone cannot explain the backlash.

Many factors contributed, including unhappy health professionals who badmouthed HMOs, the negative depiction by the media, and significant insensitivities and poor decisions by the managed care industry itself. But most important, I contend, is the fact that managed care in the American context was a form of explicit in-your-face rationing. The sense of being denied under explicit rationing is more obvious than when services are difficult to find or insurance coverage is inadequate. With explicit managed care, patients and doctors had to ask representatives of insurance companies for permission to pursue certain tests or treatments and such requests were sometimes explicitly denied, often without convincing explanations. Neither doctors nor patients liked asking, and they especially disliked being turned down, contending that medical care decisions should be left to them. As costs have escalated, some managed care strategies are being reintroduced and new ones tried.[23] American doctors and patients want to remain in the driver's seat, and their wishes are likely to affect the range of realistic future options.

Financing Increasing Expectations

The American political system, with its separation of powers and distrust of concentrated influence, provides the context in which policies in health care must be framed. While many analysts have attributed the difficulties of large-scale health reform in America to our particular governmental institutions, there are examples of vast transformations in the public sector despite these governmental barriers. Over the past several decades, for example, the United States expanded its prison systems at dizzying speed and the number of individuals incarcerated at enormous expense. One does not hear much about gridlock or stalemate in relation to these developments.[24]

Perhaps the single most important dilemma as we face our medical futures is the large and growing gap between the kind of health care Americans desire and the unwillingness of government and employers to finance the increasing bill. This dilemma will grow in intensity with increasing numbers of persons eligible for Medicare and the extraordinary growth of new technologies and treatments, aggressively marketed. The impending cost growth is not a new issue; we have worried about containing costs now for several decades. The costs of health care have continued on an upward trajectory in most years far exceeding inflation. Yet, somehow, we muddle through, although we often fail to appreciate the consequences. Some argue that more health care is a worthwhile investment, of greater value to individuals and society than most others, and that as new possibilities loom it would be acceptable to spend even 20 or 25 percent of gross national product (GNP) on health care. During recent periods of recession and a sluggish economy, the health care system continued to have significant positive growth and provide millions of jobs. Others see the unconstrained growth of health care as a dangerous trajectory pushing out more important needs and investments in education, housing, homeland security, and other areas.

Government greatly subsidizes the provision of health insurance through tax policy to the tune of an estimated federal benefit in 2004 of $188.5 billion and an additional $21 billion dollars from states.[25] The major component of this tax subsidy is for employer health contributions for workers and retirees and exemption for such contributions from usual Social Security and Medicare taxes. Smaller subsidies come through tax-free health spending in flexible spending plans. In addition, the self-employed may also deduct health benefit expenditures, and employees have additional tax benefits when their health expenditures exceed a defined threshold. Comparisons with similar estimates for 1998[26] show an average annual rate of increase of the tax subsidy of about 9 percent between 1998 and 2004.

Economists mostly agree that such subsidies are misguided for two major reasons. First, they encourage more provision and uptake of comprehensive insurance than many people would seek on their own, and many economists believe that this encourages overuse of health care in situations where these services are of marginal and perhaps even no value. Second, the most comprehensive insurance and related tax subsidies are provided to higher-paid workers who benefit disproportionately. John Sheils and Randall Haught estimated that in 2004 the lowest-paid workers (earning less than $10,000) received an average subsidy of $102 compared to a subsidy of $2,780 for those earning $100,000 or more. The regressiveness of the subsidy is shown by the fact that only 28.4 percent of the tax exemption went to the 57.5 percent of workers earning less than $50,000.[27]

While efforts have been made over many years to eliminate or modify the insurance subsidy, it continues to have strong support from employer groups and unions. They maintain that employers would be less likely to offer insurance, and workers less likely to take it up, if taxes on the costs of such benefits were required. There is, of course, a compromise possible that would only tax health insurance benefits that exceed the costs of some defined basic insurance package. Existing subsidies beyond this basic level could be redirected to provide more help in obtaining insurance for low-income employees or helping the uninsured obtain coverage. But up to now the tax subsidy has been resistant to modifications.

It is often claimed that the high cost of medical care undermines American competitiveness in world markets, but economists are mostly skeptical. The real issue, they tell us, is the cost of labor, which includes both wages and benefits. In the aggregate, they believe that workers trade off additional wages for health benefits, and employers who do not offer health insurance generally must offer higher wages. Employees, however, are less likely to see this relationship, and many tend to think of benefits independently of their wages. While correct at the aggregate level, it is difficult to demonstrate the link in individual cases, making the perception of health benefits as "free" seem plausible.

On the governmental side, the growth of the cost of entitlements and other health programs causes difficulty since there is strong public resistance to increased taxes or increased enrollee cost sharing. Medicare is financed by a designated Medicare payroll tax, enrollee premiums, and general revenues. Increased demand, coverage, or the cost of services require more resources, whether from government or enrollees. Medicaid, a shared federal-state program, has grown enormously in recent years as a proportion of state budgets, and increasingly has put pressures on other state investments such as state infrastructure and higher education. There is continuing combat between the states and the federal government about their relative fiscal responsibilities and who should have the authority to modify programs in various ways. The financial stresses on federal and state governments lead to continuing calls to reform the structure and financing of Medicare and Medicaid, and this issue will continue to take center stage in future deliberations.

The governmental battles have little salience to people when they or their family members are seriously ill. They might recognize that in the aggregate constraints are necessary and everyone can't have everything they want, but when they or their loved ones are sick they do not want these limitations applied to them. Most also believe that health care is too expensive and they should not be called upon to pay as much as they do.

Activating Consumers and Improving Quality of Care

In recent years efforts have been made to encourage competition among health plans and providers based on the belief that such competition would diminish inefficiencies and would encourage plans and providers to offer options with the mix of price and quality that consumers most want. It is also contended that more public information on performance, and well-informed consumer choices, would induce plans to give more attention to improving quality of care. At present, under common fixed-payment arrangements unadjusted for severity of illness, plans that are identified as outstanding providers of quality attract sicker patients with many more complex problems that are more costly to treat. Existing incentives encourage plans to try to recruit healthy enrollees who are unlikely to need many services and to avoid the potential enrollees who are most sick.

There is some evidence that public transparency motivates hospitals to improve quality of care. In 2002 the Joint Commission on Accreditation of Healthcare Organizations (JCAHO) required most of its accredited hospitals to submit standardized performance information and provided quarterly feedback to hospitals on their performance on eighteen indicators of quality of care for myocardial infarction, heart failure, and pneumonia. With one exception (death in hospital after myocardial infarction), all were measures of processes of care. Analyses of data from more than three thousand hospitals between 2002 and 2004 found significant improvements on fifteen of the seventeen process measures but not on the measure of heart disease deaths.[28] Such a study does not tell us whether attention to these specific areas is associated with better or worse performance on other equally important unmeasured indicators.[29]

In a Wisconsin study of 115 hospitals, reports on adverse performance in surgical and nonsurgical care and indices of care for cardiac care, knee and hip surgery, and obstetric care were used to rank hospitals as better than expected, as expected, or worse than expected. In this controlled study, user-friendly reports for some hospitals were widely disseminated to the public, while in the case of another group of hospitals, the reports were made available to the hospitals but not disseminated to the public. No reports were provided about a third group. The largest improvements over time were found in the hospitals whose performance was publicly reported, and many fewer improvements were found when there were only private reports.[30] The fewest improvements were observed in hospitals that received no reports. Depending on varying consumer subgroups studied, from 24 percent to 57 percent had seen the public report. These respondents showed significantly improved ability to identify the highly rated hospitals, even as long as two years later. There is no information, however, on whether such knowledge actually influenced patients' choices. Nevertheless, the study suggests that hospitals are concerned about their public reputations and will improve performance when public awareness of their performance is increased.

Thus policy advocates seek to encourage competition on the basis of performance by providing information to the public on the quality of care of varying plans and providers. Such consumer awareness, they believe, will induce plans to focus more on performance issues, as the Wisconsin study suggests. In the last decade or two, significant advances have been made in measuring outcomes of medical care and establishing evidence-based standards, but their broad acceptance in everyday practice is limited. The impediments are substantial. Medical care, as extensive as it is, remains a highly decentralized activity in which local markets and local practice norms predominate. Efforts to develop credible, agreed-upon evidence-based standards are undermined by the numerous groups who wish to promulgate standards most consistent with their own interests, for example, clinical specialties who want their most remunerative interventions encouraged, pharmaceutical companies who want their drugs used, or medical device manufacturers who want their products promoted. Thus, there is a proliferation of practice standards from many different organizations. Many medical organizations have become highly dependent on the pharmaceutical and other medical industries for support.[31] Participants developing practice guidelines often have serious conflicts of interest.

As noted earlier, an effort by the Agency for Health Care Policy and Research in the early 1990s to develop guidelines in important areas of care, based on the best evidence, led to significant budget reductions and almost led to the elimination of the agency.[32] It became evident that developing guidelines in the American political environment was a hazardous endeavor, and the government removed itself from the practice guideline business. This is not true of some other countries, where government agencies seek to establish what interventions are cost-effective and what should be covered. For example, the National Institute for Clinical Excellence (NICE) in England (recently renamed the National Institute for Health and Clinical Excellence) assesses various treatments and makes recommendations on coverage to the

National Health Service. Even in England this is a contentious activity that results in much criticism and controversy, but NICE appears to have greater credibility and public acceptance than similar efforts in the United States. The Medicare program in the United States makes such determinations, but the process is subjected to great external pressures, and Congress often interferes.

It is inevitable that public entitlement programs move in this direction, and a significant step was taken in the Medicare Prescription Drug, Improvement, and Modernization Act of 2003. Section 1013 of this act directs the secretary of the Department of Health and Human Services (HSS) to conduct and support research on "the outcomes, comparative clinical effectiveness, and appropriateness of health care items and services (including prescription drugs)" and to establish a process "to develop priorities that will guide the research, demonstrations and evaluation activities." The act also calls for the synthesis of scientific evidence "with respect to the comparative clinical effectiveness, outcomes, appropriateness, and provision of such items and services (including prescription drugs)," noting the inclusion of items that impose a high cost as well as overutilized and underutilized services. Section 1013 is seen as an effort to make patients more discerning consumers by providing them with easily understood information. It also mandates broad and ongoing consultation with stakeholders in setting research priorities. Section 1013 treads quite carefully in the minefields of special interests, requiring the director of the Agency for Healthcare Research and Quality to "not mandate national standards of clinical practice or quality health care standards" and to advertise this prohibition when reporting recommendations.

It is challenging to induce patients to make medical care decisions on the basis of indicators of effectiveness. In recent years much effort has been made to develop indicators for report cards that allow comparisons among health plans, hospitals, medical groups, and even among some specialist physicians such as cardiovascular surgeons. Some indicators are now routinely reported for HMOs, health plans, and nursing homes by the federal government, some state health departments, and a variety of private organizations. Although the indicators available are simply a small sample among the many services and procedures performed, they provide some useful information that patients can use to make choices. Advocates of managed competition would like to have consumers use such indicators of quality to select health plans and providers as a way of incentivizing the system to compete on the basis of quality of performance as well as on cost.

Progress in getting consumers to use such information meaningfully has been slow. Most do not use such available information in making health care choices and regard most sources of such information as having limited credibility. Health plans and the media have low credibility for providing such advice, and, perhaps surprisingly, patients have little trust in government advice as well. As in the past, patients prefer what is most familiar and the advice of people they believe have no ulterior motives in advising them. Thus, they give high credibility to the advice of relatives and friends, their personal physicians, and other health professionals they know personally. When asked to choose hypothetically between a hospital familiar to them and one recommended by experts, the majority of patients choose the familiar.[33] Personal physicians have great influence on their patents' choices and in most instances make these choices for them.

We face the significant challenge of developing credible and authoritative referees who can inform the health professional community and the public of what is known about important medical modalities, the cost-effectiveness of alternative interventions, and the quality of care and outcomes achieved by various provider groups. While Section 1013 tends in this direction, it in itself will not lead to the necessary authoritative voice, which will require active professional, public, and private collaboration and protection from political interference. We also need credible institutions to consider what is fair care allocation and how decisions can be made in ways that are respectful of reasonable differences of opinion.[34] Meeting these challenges will involve important technical issues as well as sensitive political ones. Much remains uncertain, and this makes it even more essential that we have institutions that can promote impartial assessments and build public and patient trust. Efforts are being made within large, organized practices to introduce practice guidelines for meaningful case management in such important chronic conditions as diabetes, asthma, heart failure, and depression. Through the use of nurse practitioners and effective teamwork, supported by electronic medical records and the use of prompts and reminders, quality of care can be improved. Focusing thoughtful efforts on high-risk patients can reduce costly acute episodes.[35]

The United States has an impressive research and development infrastructure, admirable scientific accomplishments, excellent institutions of higher education and professional preparation, and high levels of technical innovation. Studies of quality and outcomes find, however, that care is commonly deficient; as much as 50 percent of recommended care is not provided,[36] wasteful and inappropriate care is common, and medical and hospital errors abound, resulting in many deaths and injuries.[37] These errors are often due not to incompetent and negligent professionals, although such exist, but to poorly designed systems of care that increase the probability of error and accident. The challenge is to take what we know and design practice systems and organizational procedures that make it possible to detect impending problems and avoid mistakes. Such organizational understanding exists and has proven useful in improving many care settings. We have to implement these systems more widely.

Issues of Trust

Given the required trade-offs and the many uncertainties as we try to achieve a more coherent system of care, it is important to have credible spokespersons who can help the public understand its options. In earlier times the medical profession had the public's confidence, but it no longer speaks with one voice or has high credibility. Nor has government much credibility, and the public's respect for authority and expertise has generally very much eroded. This is a worldwide phenomenon across all sectors including medicine, which for much of the twentieth century was insulated from distrust because of the reverence that many had for their personal physicians. While trust in one's personal physician is still quite strong, distrust in medical leadership is now on par with distrust in other institutional leadership in government and the private sector. The majority of the public do not necessarily anticipate that their medical leaders will work in their interests.[38]

The loss of confidence in leadership is characteristic of a mass society with many channels of information and communication. News reaches people immediately from all over the world, and the media focus on disagreement and conflict, betrayals of trust, and competing points of view. Thus, people gain the impression that the morals and trustworthiness of their leaders are less than in past times. More specifically, in the case of medical care, the media expose the population to disagreements about treatment and care, conflicts among specialists, the uncertainty of medical evidence, and stories about medical errors and poor-quality care. Thus, much of the public is skeptical about leaving health care decisions to medical leaders. They trust their chosen personal physicians, but that trust diminishes when they see their physicians constrained by larger institutional controls. Although it has been documented repeatedly that fee-for-service medicine contributes to overutilization, patients seem less concerned about unnecessary treatment than the possibility that something of value may be withheld. Patients are reluctant to accept that treatments they have learned about from direct-to-consumer advertising or from friends are unneeded, and physicians are faced by time pressures that make detailed explanations difficult. Unwilling to alienate their patients, doctors often give them what they wish. The media are an important part of this process and contribute to raising patients' insecurities and demands.

Individual or Population Health

Medical care is in its provision an individualized endeavor focused on treating people one at a time. Doctors are trained to think of themselves as advocates first and foremost for the interests of each individual patient they treat, and such patient advocacy is central to what patients seek from their doctors. Although there is much concern about the need to use medical resources prudently and take account of the needs of the entire community, patients want their doctors to focus on their needs and put their interests before all else. A vigorous debate continues about whether physicians have responsibilities that go beyond their individual patients, and whether making trade-offs that take others into account is an ethical professional stance.

A vigorous debate also persists at the societal level about the massive resources devoted to curing specific diseases relative to the much smaller resources devoted to prevention and health promotion. Medical care is increasingly important to health and longevity, but its influence remains modest relative to the other forces that shape health. Many factors influence the health of community populations, including the material and social circumstances of people's lives, their work and family situations and social supports, the quality of parenting and children's social development, nutrition, patterns of living and exposure to toxins and other environmental risks, exposure to infections and epidemics, and damaging health and social behaviors. Environment interacts in complex ways with genetic endowment and biology, beginning in utero and continuing over the entire life course. Many individuals believe that we would do well to allocate a larger proportion of our health investments to public and population health initiatives. Compassion and empathy are typically quite individual, however, and the public responds more to the identifiable patient in distress than to abstract ideas about preventable diseases and deaths in large populations.

Nevertheless, policy initiatives and interventions designed to influence the environmental exposures and behaviors of populations can have large influence on health. It is valuable to work with individuals to reduce abuse of substances, improve nutrition, and reduce exposure to infectious diseases, but policy actions that affect drug use, guns, the food industry, release of toxic substances into the environment, and many other aspects of living can have large impact on health trends across large populations. Impediments to community action include push-back from special interests who benefit from current arrangements. Much that could be done is left undone at the community level.

The Course Ahead

The larger context of American values, political institutions, and politics sets the opportunities and constraints for alternative ways to restructure the components of health care so that they can function as parts of a more rational system. The focus on our failures to achieve a national health insurance program sometimes masks the extent to which our system has undergone continuing transformations in financing, organization, and performance. While some critics see the politics of health as "dynamics without change,"[39] the system of care has been adaptive, innovative, and resilient in many ways. At the governmental levels, Medicare, Medicaid, the state Children's Health Insurance Program, the Department of Veterans Affairs (VA), and the Federal Employees Health Benefits Program have covered the needs of a wide range of the population and have evolved over time in many innovative ways.

Change in the American health care system tends to come in smaller iterations where opposing worldviews are less salient, where outcomes are less defined and more uncertain, where many groups see possible changes serving their interests, and where compromise is more possible. Big reform ideas usually engage much of the public and lobbying organizations and become highly politicized, making change extremely difficult. But much policy in the health care system is highly technical, does not engage the interest of the larger public or even the media, and is worked out in private deliberations by powerful political figures, activists who have large interests at stake, lobbyists, and technical experts.[40] Seemingly small and boring decisions such as how much Medicare will pay for particular medical procedures, how depreciation on capital expenditures will be handled, how different professionals will be paid, and how tax law will be applied can have large influence on many aspects of care, such as capital investment in facilities, the provision of health services, and the willingness of employers to provide insurance to their employees. There is little transparency in these seemingly small policy matters, but their various iterations come to shape your health care and mine. Most Americans probably know little if anything about the Balanced Budget Amendment (BBA) of 1997, but this omnibus budget reconciliation bill has had large reverberations throughout much of our health care system. Many more Americans are familiar with one aspect of the BBA, the part that established the state Children's Health Insurance Program, a major initiative with the states that provided coverage to uninsured children and cushioned the loss of insurance experienced by many children following welfare reform.

The financing of American health care runs the gamut from traditional fee-for-service to capitation and prospective payment and many blended schemes. In the private and provider sectors we have seen extraordinary innovation and change as health plans and professionals combine and recombine in various ways to take advantage of new innovations, capture market share, and gain bargaining leverage.[41] American health care offers every conceivable arrangement. This is of course untidy and makes it difficult to impose meaningful rationality. Those who are lucky may indeed get the best care available anywhere, but overall our system yields much confusion, waste, and poor value for money.

Most people who have thought carefully about health care understand that if we are to reach our health goals and reduce inequalities we must have universal coverage that provides everyone with basic care. They also understand that doing everything technically possible for everyone would break the bank. Provision of care must be contained in meaningful ways, and trade-offs are necessary. Providers now often face incentives that encourage more expensive rather than less expensive treatments of little added value, and patients are often deceived about the value of treatments and drugs by misleading promotion. But no one doubts the powerful forces against constraints. The challenges we face are awesome, and all indications are that conditions may get worse in the years ahead. In the chapters that follow, I address a range of these issues and the initiatives required to direct American health care in more constructive directions.

Chapter 2

What Is Disease and
What Should We Treat?

A major challenge to the financing and organization of health care is the continuing medicalization of the problems of everyday life. The definition of disease has always been a bit murky, tied to social, religious, and moral ideologies about desirable and undesirable behavior, with a tendency to characterize many behaviors that violated current social norms as sick. The debates, for example, about whether masturbation, homosexuality, and promiscuous behavior were diseases waxed and waned over the years as cultural ideas changed, but persons engaged in these behaviors were given many so-called treatments and were even institutionalized. With greater enlightenment we might believe that this is a problem of the past and that good science now reigns, but, if anything, the ambiguities of disease definition are compounded. In an age of ever changing ideas and technologies, it is increasingly difficult to establish any kind of consensus on what is and is not illness.

The tasks of identifying illness and providing appropriate treatment have layers of complexity. Many different groups seek to impose their definitions on the health care system, on the need for treatment, and on what insurers must pay for. They attempt to influence public demand, physician and institutional behavior, and social policies affecting the provision of care. In one sense the health system is a free-for-all in which many different forces try to promote their views of what constitutes risk and disease, what the health system should be, and what it should provide. Patients buy into some concepts and not others; different professionals, medical specialties, scientists, alternative practitioners, advocacy groups, pundits, and policy makers are all part of the mix. The result is a bit of a moving target, always in at least a partial state of chaos. Many aspire to a more unified, predictable, and stable system of care; others view its dynamic messiness and its flexibility in accommodating diverse constituencies as a source of innovation.

How Biology and Environment Shape Need

The more we learn about human biology the clearer it becomes that people are highly adaptive to their environments including climate, sources of food and nutrition, altitude and air quality, and much more. Our biologies are also highly responsive to the social and cultural context and patterns of social relationships, work, and family life. In the larger sense, organisms adapt over time in a Darwinian sense through natural selection and the survival of traits that better fit environmental challenges. But even in the very short run, organisms must accommodate to rapid environmental, cultural, and social change. Health care as an instrument of culture seeks to facilitate adaptation and sustain individuals and groups as they cope with their own limitations and changing environments and cultures.

The ageless arguments about whether biology or environment are more important now seem much less relevant as we understand better that genetic endowments are not static and that expressed traits depend importantly on how biological propensities and environment interact. One of the areas, for example, where the nature/nurture argument has been contentious has been in the study of depression, where social and genetic determinists have argued vehemently but for the most part have talked past one another. A recent analysis of stressful life events and the serotonin transporter (5-HT T) gene in depression illustrates a more productive line of inquiry. This longitudinal, prospective study of a birth cohort of 1,037 children in Dunedin, New Zealand, assessed many times beginning at age three and followed-up at age twenty-six, examined the role of life stress among individuals with one or two copies of the short allele of this gene.[1] At the aggregate level the study found, as have many others, that persons under high stress are more likely to become clinically depressed. However, it was primarily persons with one or two copies of the short allele who were susceptible to the clinical condition under stress. Those with short alleles were unlikely to become depressed in the absence of significant stress. Those who had both alleles of the long kind were protected even when experiencing comparably high stress. The hypothesis that biological propensities are triggered by stress is not new; in fact, it has been perhaps the most commonly held understanding among stress researchers. But the study shows impressively the value of understanding how both biology and environment interact, and suggests how prevention efforts might be better targeted.

We have come to understand dysfunctional and harmful bodily states through the medical disease model, a pragmatic tool that has served society well in identifying pathology and developing beneficial interventions. The disease model seeks to identify clusters of symptoms and signs that have a coherent identity and that represent an underlying disorder. Depending on the state of knowledge, identifying the disorder correctly provides information on its likely course over time, its causes, and its appropriate treatment. When a disease is well understood, making a correct diagnosis opens a flood of useful information and guidance. If the diagnosis is incorrect, it usually takes doctor and patient down the wrong path. The disease diagnosis is basically a theory. Its utility in any case depends on the degree of confirmation and the degree to which there are effective treatments.[2] A diagnosis of pernicious anemia provides excellent guidance about treatment. A diagnosis of chronic fatigue syndrome provides very little.

A significant characteristic of the medical disease model is that it is creates dichotomies; people are said to either have or not have a disorder. But many biological functions are continua, and each one's value on the continuum may or may not be adaptive to the environment depending on its specific demands. The Aymara Indians in the Peruvian Andes, living in high altitudes with less oxygen, have much greater lung capacity and blood rich in hemoglobin than persons unadapted to high altitudes.[3] So whether lung capacity is adequate depends on demands of the environment and prior adaptations. Many of the major indicators used in medicine such as blood pressure and blood lipid values are continua with considerable range of differences in populations. Persons are said to have the disease known as hypertension when blood pressure reaches a threshold value, most traditionally 140 systolic and 90 diastolic. Epidemiological studies have documented that while high blood pressure is asymptomatic in most cases, persons who exceed this threshold are more prone to heart attacks, stroke, other damage to organs, and premature death, and this justifies intervention. Studies also show, however, that blood pressure in relation to risk is more linear than a dichotomous approach implies and that risk grows as blood pressure increases.[4] From a risk point of view, lower blood pressure within limits is better. The threshold for initiating treatments to lower blood pressure depends on assessments of the magnitude of risks, the costs of lifetime treatment, and the difficulties of keeping asymptomatic persons on a lifetime drug regimen. In recent years it has been argued that persons with marginally high blood pressure should be treated. As points lower on the distribution are chosen and become close to average values of blood pressure in the population, the potentially treatable population becomes very large.[5] Simply focusing on high-risk individuals will miss the majority of persons who subsequently have heart attacks and strokes, but it is extraordinarily expensive to treat everyone. Nor do we understand the long-term consequences.

Similar considerations are increasingly common in other areas of treatment. Studies suggest that the use of statins in treating low density lipoproteins (LDL) reduces risk of heart attacks, and persons of relatively average risk increasingly are being treated. Some British investigators have advocated that all people over age fifty-five take a polypill containing a statin, three hypertensives, folic acid, and aspirin, as a way of preventing heart attacks.[6] Depressive symptoms below the threshold of a diagnosis of clinical depression are now commonly treated with selective serotonin uptake inhibitors (SSRIs). Such depressive symptoms could be distressing and disabling, but the value of such treatment has not been established. We will explore the implications of mass preventive treatment in later consideration of how best to promote population health.

The definitions of what is disease and what constitutes risk are arbitrary, depending on opinions about harm. Generally, we become concerned with body states when they contribute importantly to discomfort, disability, or expected future harm. But many behaviors and personal attributes that cause pain and threaten harm are not diseases. Many jobs, sports activities, and social behaviors may involve high risk of danger and harm, but involvement in such activities is valued and not seen as relevant to medical concern. In addition to potential harmfulness, it is usually assumed that a disease or disorder is in some sense a dysfunction of the organism; it is not the way the organism is understood to function. The heart is normally expected to pump blood adequately to the various tissues and cells, the kidneys to appropriately regulate fluids, the ears to hear, and so on. When these processes break down they are dysfunctions. Similar considerations apply to behavior. Engaging in dangerous sports is viewed as normal from a cultural perspective; standing in the middle of major highways dodging cars is not and implies that some important mental function has become impaired. But it is not inconceivable that a subculture could develop in some subgroups of young, risk-taking individuals who adopt this seemingly bizarre behavior as a "cool sport." Such entertainments as illegal sideshows in which youth gather late at night on city streets while drivers swing their cars into doughnuts and other figures and street racing exemplify such subcultures.

This is all messy enough, but there are further complications. Many of the constellations of symptoms called diseases are not scientifically validated syndromes but simply informed judgments about symptoms that are empirically associated. Most of the disease definitions in the *Diagnostic and Statistical Manual of the American Psychiatric Association* (DSM-IV) are simply committee judgments of appropriate thresholds to characterize the clinical relevance of symptom groupings and have no independent validity. These characterizations of disorder serve as conveniences for research, professional communication, reimbursement, and other social judgments, but they are unconfirmed in any scientific sense against independent markers. Many interests work to define and gain acceptance of new diseases and the adoption of new treatments. Manufacturers of pharmaceuticals and other products seek to develop markets; they do so by defining new conditions that might benefit from their products. Medical specialties have developed around definitions of disease that fit new medical and surgical technologies and interventions and provide remunerative practice niches. Patient advocates organize to promote acceptance of diagnoses and causation concepts that frame their problems in particular ways, reduce stigmatization of them, and legitimize reimbursement from private and public payers. Patient groups have organized around such entities as Lyme disease, chemical sensitivity disorders, and chronic fatigue to make their problems more central to public awareness and to elicit public and medical acceptance. The National Alliance for the Mentally Ill built its advocacy around the theme that mental illnesses were disorders of the brain, not simply psychological and social maladjustments.

An additional layer of complication comes from patients themselves, who have their own ideas of what constitutes illness and what problems require medical intervention. Patients have varying inclinations to perceive and define symptoms, to define them in particular ways, to give them attention, to seek lay or professional assistance, to seek help from one or another type of practitioner, and to cooperate in treatment. The field of study dealing with these patterns is called illness behavior. Many influences shape the perceptions and responses of patients, including their early experience and upbringing, their experience with illness, the particular cultural and social ideas they are exposed to within their social context, their level of education and scientific literacy, their interest in health issues, and their exposure to the media. Patients also have different sensitivities to bodily indications and to pain and discomfort, influenced in part by biological propensities, by social learning, and by the norms and demands of their immediate social context. Reaction to pain is an exemplary way to illustrate how a biological phenomenon is influenced by subjective factors, including social norms about expressing distress and people's beliefs about the importance of stoicism.[7] These factors influence not only what people express but also the meanings they attribute to inner states and what they experience. Henry Beecher, a distinguished Harvard anesthesiologist, observed many years ago that injured soldiers evacuated from combat situations complained less of pain than civilian surgical patients with much less body trauma. Beecher interpreted these varying responses in terms of contrasting meanings attributed to their situations by soldiers returning to safety as compared with civilians facing fearful interventions.[8]

It is difficult to say what is illness and what it is not in this conglomeration of influences. Traditionally, medicine skirted the issue by treating anyone coming to doctors with complaints as legitimate. Occasionally, chronically complaining patients who would not accept reassurance were labeled by doctors as hypochondriacs, or more invidiously as "crocks" or "turkeys," but doctors had an interest in keeping their fee-for-service patients happy. Studies repeatedly found that most people had symptoms at any given time that credibly could be presented in medical settings, given a diagnosis, and treated in some fashion. In a classic study in 1961, Kerr White, T. Franklin Williams, and Bernard Greenberg analyzed data from various population surveys. They estimated that in any given month 75 percent of the population had one or more illnesses or injuries, although only one of three of these people consulted a physician.[9] The surveys underestimated the actual occurrence of symptoms; most of these surveys only counted as symptoms those that people did something about.[10] Forty years later Larry Green and his colleagues used the 1996 Medical Expenditure Panel Survey to make comparable types of estimates.[11] They found that 80 percent of survey respondents reported symptoms each month, 33 percent considered seeking medical care, and 22 percent visited a physician. Many different types of factors determine who among those with symptoms seeks care, including social and cultural characteristics, perceived severity of the illness and the extent it interfered with functioning, insurance coverage, availability of a personal physician, and the accessibility and convenience involved in receiving care. Although seriousness of illness is one of the more important predictors, some patients with very serious illness fail to seek care while others with relatively minor symptoms seek care readily.

When epidemiologists study illness at the population level, where persons' self-definition of whether they are ill is less relevant and independent judgments of illness and risk are made, investigators usually depend on measuring reported symptoms, impairments, measures from various tests and procedures, and the like. There may be significant discrepancy between perceived symptoms and subjective health assessment and test results. Many persons, for example, who on imaging have seeming abnormalities of their spine may experience no discomfort, while others who complain of chronic discomfort have no such signs.[12] Similar lack of correspondence between objective measures and subjective responses are common for many other problems, such as gastrointestinal complaints and headache. In counting cases, epidemiologists prefer medical assessments confirmed by objective measures and independent tests. When these do not exist, as in the case of many mental disorders, epidemiologists commonly use measures that take account of impairments associated with symptoms to assess the burden of disease and whether it requires intervention.

When patients paid directly for their care the issue of who sought varying types of care was of limited social importance. In American society persons are free to spend their disposable income as they wish, and those who preferred more medical care to alternative expenditures did little harm. Under contemporary conditions, however, most people have health insurance coverage and excessive use affects everyone's premiums. Also, taxpayers in one way or another pay much of the bill, so frivolous and unnecessary uses have social relevance. Moreover, medical technologies can be harmful, so misuse of care, whether by patients' choices or physicians' decisions, has important consequences. It is no longer viable to support whatever patients demand and whatever physicians are willing to provide, if it ever was. We need more sophisticated ways of determining need and appropriate care. We probably would not want to be restrictive for less expensive visits that are important to patients in providing information, support, and reassurance, but we have to think carefully about the expensive and invasive technologies and treatments that some patients demand and that may involve serious risks.

How, then, do we structure a system that allocates care appropriately to those who need it? It is prudent to allow people who are uncertain about their health status to receive an informed assessment. Having a primary care clinician who treats most ordinary conditions and provides overall guidance to a patient about further care is the way health problems are typically handled in most of the world. The United States is a bit of an exception because its medical system is greatly tilted toward specialist care, but even here most patients have a personal doctor who functions as a primary care provider.

Two competing theories on how best to make decisions about need and care reflect the broad ideological division between marketplace advocates and those who favor planned systems with more central control. Among marketplace advocates, patient cost sharing is seen as the most efficient way to fit the provision of medical care to need and patient preferences. Such cost sharing occurs at two levels. At the insurance level, these advocates argue that persons should be able to select insurance coverage at different levels of financial risk and cost sharing. They argue that those who prefer more than standard coverage should be able to obtain it but should pay the difference between the true cost and some established standard cost that constitutes an appropriate health insurance subsidy by employers or government. Thus, for example, employees who have a choice of plans and select the more expensive traditional indemnity plan should pay the additional cost between that and a defined basic plan. There are many versions of these proposals, some of which would provide rebates to those who select less than standard care, such as only catastrophic coverage, but the basic underlying idea is similar. Those who want more than standard coverage would be expected to pay extra for it.

At the more immediate service level, market advocates believe that co-insurance, that is, patients sharing the costs of services they use, encourages them to be more prudent buyers of care relative to need and to seek services they really believe have value. But this may exaggerate patient control, since physicians make most of the expensive treatment decisions without significant patient input. Co-insurance that puts people at high cost-sharing risk (95 percent of cost up to some threshold amount such as $1,000 per family) as compared with care with no co-insurance reduced the demand for ambulatory care by about a quarter in the only randomized experiment ever done on this issue.[13] There are two major difficulties with such cost-sharing approaches. First, they influence the behavior of persons with low incomes differently from persons with higher incomes, encouraging inequities in care that many people believe are inappropriate. This could be minimized by subsidies to persons with lower incomes. More serious, however, is that co-insurance is a very crude barrier to care that filters out both trivial and useful care. People don't necessarily know when they could benefit from treatment. Thus, co-insurance results in the provision of less appropriate and efficacious care than would be desirable. Moreover, this deficiency is most likely to be experienced by persons with less education and income, who have more illness but less health knowledge and sophistication.

A more recent version of the market idea and making consumers more prudent purchasers is the idea of consumer-driven health plans (CDHPs), an idea strongly encouraged by Republicans and the Bush administration as a means of controlling the growth of health care expenditures. CDHPs involve combining high-deductible health insurance with tax-advantaged spending accounts. There are now a variety of these tax-privileged instruments, but the Health Savings Account (HSA) is particularly being promoted as an alternative to more traditional insurance coverage. The enrollee must acquire a high-deductible health plan with at least a $1,000 deductible for single coverage ($1,000 to $5,000) and $2,000 for family coverage ($2,000 to $10,000). Employers and/or employees can make pre-tax contributions up to a specified limit to a HSA, and the enrollee who owns this fund uses it to pay front end health care costs. The enrollee has the advantage of tax-free deposits and interest and tax-free withdrawals when the money is used for qualified medical expenses. Unused funds can be carried over from year to year and are portable when a person moves to a new job or retires. In any year, there is a ceiling for out-of-pocket costs; in 2004 the ceiling was $5,000 for oneself and $10,000 for family coverage.

The logic of the HSA is that persons are now spending their own money, not the money of the insurance company, and thus will be motivated to make more prudent choices using increasingly available public information about cost and quality of health services. Since recent legislation has made these plans more advantageous, more employers seem to be offering the option, and there has been significant growth in enrollment. These plans are attractive to young, healthy people who have few serious health care needs; they offer few advantages to people with chronic disease who can anticipate higher use of health care services. Some of these plans come with various bells and whistles such as exclusion of some preventive treatments from deductibles to encourage the use of such services.

Consumer-driven health plans and health savings accounts have all the previously discussed advantages and disadvantages of co-insurance and deductibles. They set up a psychological barrier to using basic health services, particularly among persons with less income, on the assumption that they really know when they need and can benefit from care. While some trivial use is probably prevented, some useful services inevitably are also screened out. Since these plans are likely to be more attractive to the healthy than to the sick, it remains unclear whether they limit costs significantly, or even whether people can wisely use available information to make thoughtful and prudent health choices, or that these plans can reasonably constrain the more expensive diagnostic and treatment decisions made by physicians. Persons with serious illness are likely to exceed the deductible, and most medical costs are incurred by a small proportion of the public. Thus, the expected containment of costs through such plans is unlikely. Moreover, the multiplicity of these plans is likely to add significantly to administrative costs. From a broader social point of view, these plans undermine the idea of sharing risk by removing healthy people with low expected expenses from the larger insurance pool, making traditional health insurance more costly for those with serious illness.

While some people welcome the idea of not subsidizing others, segmenting the risk pool undermines social solidarity and the idea that we as a nation share advantages and adversities.

An alternative approach to control costs is to use some of the strategies characteristic of managed care and some universal health care plans in other countries. Such health insurance programs make it relatively easy for patients to enter the health system through their primary care clinician but then use various controls to manage more intensive uses of care. In these systems, the primary care doctor functions as a gatekeeper to more expensive specialty care and other expensive interventions, and patients are less able to refer themselves directly to these services. Also, because these practices are part of systems, and under more managerial control, they are more able to put in place quality-assurance processes, practice incentives, and cost constraints that are difficult to impose within traditional fee-for-service practice. Other ways of constraining costs in these systems include limitations on supply of specialists and technologies, drug formularies, and noncoverage of services that fail to meet evidence-based standards.

Capitation payment (the provision of a predetermined fixed payment per patient per unit of time) or fixed prospective payment for a diagnosis (as in hospital prospective payment in the Medicare PPS program) or for an entire care episode (as is common in obstetrics) encourages the provider to be efficient and to restrain use of unnecessary or minimally beneficial services. Capitation has the opposite risk of fee-for-service. Fee-for-service may encourage use of services of marginal or no value, or more expensive treatments than needed, because they are remunerative for the provider. Capitation, in contrast, may encourage withholding some useful and appropriate services. The hope is that medical professionalism will moderate such tendencies, but much in medicine is uncertain and at the margins payment incentives influence decision making. The different weaknesses of fee-for-service and capitation feed into the opposing positions of market advocates and those who support a more planned system.

The central issue is how to organize an approach to health care provision that is affordable, excludes no one, and offers the best opportunity to respond meaningfully to need. Open-ended and well-financed systems, as in the United States, may provide much care, but they are not organized to distribute such care to best meet population needs. Too much basic care of value, such as immunizations and treatments for hypertension, diabetes, depression, and other serious conditions, is not adequately provided, while expensive and untested treatments often are promoted and excessively used. Given how need comes to be defined, responsibility rests with patients as well as clinicians. This suggests the importance of patient education, a serious alliance between clinician and patient, and organizational systems that monitor the status of patients and communicate to them what they and the medical system can do together to best meet their needs and avoid future illness and disability.

Developing such an effective doctor-patient alliance may require more time than doctors are likely to give, or that insurers or patients are likely to be willing to pay for adequately. It is estimated that a serious patient/doctor partnership requires about half an hour for a primary care visit. This time expectation seems unrealistic, but new information technologies and disease-management approaches make such partnerships more viable.[14] A well-organized electronic medical record allows medical practices to monitor their patient populations, develop disease registries, identify unmet needs, provide prompts and reminders to clinicians and patients, promote evidence-based standards of care, and keep track of drug interactions and contra indications. There is growing evidence that disease-management systems for chronic diseases such as heart failure, depression, asthma, and diabetes, in which nurses and educators play a major role relieving the workload of physicians, can provide good and timely care and counseling that prevents expensive avoidable problems and emergencies and improves patients' quality of life. There will always be failures to respond appropriately to need because of patient, clinician, and system factors. Patients often have complicated and difficult lives, many responsibilities, too little time, and other limited resources, and they may find cooperation too difficult and expected regimens inconsistent with their life routines. Clinicians may be rushed and feel overwhelmed, and may lack the time, inclination, or understanding to devise treatment approaches that fit patients' social and personal needs. Many system and practice factors that could either facilitate or inhibit appropriate care may not be easily modified by individual clinicians, and they cope as best they can. Managers may understand the value of new information technologies and disease-management approaches that are promoted as ways to identify high-risk persons early and intervene before episodes become crises, but they remain skeptical as to whether such innovations really reduce cost or whether the needed investment in technology is remunerative.

Agreeing on the need for care and providing appropriate interventions are more difficult in some areas of care than others. Patients experiencing pain and incapacity are much more motivated to seek care and cooperate in treatment than those who are asymptomatic or face more distant threats such as those with high blood pressure, high cholesterol, or excess weight. Moreover, patients without symptoms are often reluctant to embark on expensive long-term treatment that may have side effects and whose future benefits are uncertain. Persons with conditions that are stigmatized, such as those with mental illnesses and substance abuse disorders, may deny a need for care, want to deal with their problems on their own, or have little trust that the medical system has much to offer them.[15] This is the case, for example, in major depression, where only a minority of those who it is believed could benefit seek or accept treatment.[16] Patient resistance and poor medical responsiveness combine in the treatment of behavioral problems, particularly substance abuse problems, where relatively few who need treatment receive it and treatment failure is common. Whether these areas are appropriately seen as medical problems and whether alternative remedial efforts are more useful also remain in dispute. Deep-seated values and beliefs about will, personal responsibility, and attitudes toward medicine overlay care in these areas.

In sum, identifying and responding to need is not simply a technical scientific endeavor. What are construed as diseases and disorders, what are viewed as valuable outcomes, and what are seen as legitimate interventions are all shaped by cultural understandings and mass media, and by the promotional activities of profit-seeking industries, the entrepreneurial motivation of health professionals, and the activities of health advocacy groups. Different coalitions and alliances form, depending on the issue. Many advocates repeatedly point to gaps in care, failures to respond to need, and instances of extraordinary neglect. Others see Americans as health absorbed, pampered, and obsessed with interventions to maintain youth, remake their bodies, and enhance their capacities. There is truth in both these characterizations, and both reflect the many ways the society and culture shape our aspirations and behavior.

Chapter 3

Saving Lives Individually or in Populations

Health and mortality vary dramatically from one place to other, reflecting social and cultural context even more than biological factors. We might ask, for example, why men in Chicago are thirty times more likely to perpetrate a homicide than men in England and Wales.[1] The overall trends in both contexts are similar. Both have much lower risk among women, rising risk in youth and young adulthood, and declining risk in older age. But the cross-national differences in prevalence dwarf all else. We can spend a great deal of money looking for a gene for violence, and biological factors undoubtedly contribute something to our overall understanding of violence, but if we are looking to reduce the murder rate we better be looking elsewhere.

It has long been understood that the health of populations is shaped by many determinants, from agriculture and food production to the control of infectious disease through sanitation, assurance of water quality, appropriate public health structures, and other factors. Historical demographers debate the relative importance of nutrition, standards of living, and governmental institutional arrangements among other factors, but there is consensus that, at least historically, the role of medical care, in contrast to public health, has had limited influence on mortality.[2]

This has changed in the last several decades. In the United States, for example, increased life expectancy and certainly the quality of life among older Americans are substantially attributable to advances in medicine and medical technology.[3] Similarly, the more recent decline in infant deaths and the survival of low-birth-weight babies are largely a result of new sophisticated medical technologies.[4] Unfortunately, infants of very low birth weight who are kept alive by technology have many more chronic conditions, functional limitations, and continuing dependency needs in later life than infants of normal birth weight.[5] The most dramatic advance in the last several decades has been the decline in mortality from cardiovascular disease, and impressively among men who faced the greatest risks. The fall in heart disease mortality is still not fully explained, and not so easily attributable to changes in individual health behavior as some maintain, but it is clear that part of this improvement is due to new pharmaceuticals, cardiovascular surgery, and other medical responses.[6] Medical care appears now to have a larger role in affecting longevity and improvements in health than in the past, but broader social determinants continue to explain most of the variations in patterns of mortality and disease.

We devote the vast majority of our health resources to medical care of individuals and relatively little to preventive efforts at the community level. Approximately half the deaths in the United States each year can be attributed to a limited number of behaviors and environmental exposures, including smoking, poor diets, and limited physical activity.[7]

Two decades ago Geoffrey Rose, an eminent British epidemiologist, brought to professional awareness the important distinction between interventions focused on sick individuals and those focused on sick populations.[8] Although these approaches are not in opposition, they have different implications for how we choose to make investments in health interventions. The focus on individuals largely involves a risk factor approach in which persons who face health risks are identified and efforts made to intervene through education, medications, and behavior changes. Familiar examples are efforts to help individuals give up smoking and improve their diets and exercise routines, or taking medications to reduce risk factors associated with disease, such as blood pressure and cholesterol. The population approach is less obvious and requires more detailed discussion.

Risk factor differences among individuals are easy to identify when there are large variations on the relevant measures within the population studied. However, populations may be relatively homogeneous on important risk factors, and thus risks to population health may not be fully apparent. If everyone in a geographic area is subjected to comparable levels of environmental pollutants, diets high in fat, inactive lifestyles, or hundreds of other conditions that affect health, we may not fully appreciate the significance of these factors in generating important health outcomes. By studying factors across population groups we can better appreciate some of the major determinants of population health and the extent to which varying environments either promote health or increase risks of disease.

Think again about the homicide difference between Chicago and England and Wales. Clearly, we can learn some useful things by studying differences in risks of homicide in Chicago. Simply focusing on Chicago, however, fails to explain much of the variation between Chicago and England and Wales. Or to take a different kind of example, why is hypertension, common in developed countries, less common in some African societies, and why does blood pressure increase with age in developed countries but not in all societies?[9] When we ask such questions we are no longer talking about individual risk but, in contrast, about population averages and what we might do in a more global way to change them. We know that there are many individual factors associated with harmful blood lipid levels, from genetics to individual behavior, but if we want to understand why Finland has had such high levels of coronary heart disease and Japan such low levels, we have to go beyond individuals, and examine such things as culture, diet, food distribution, and normative patterns of behavior.

As Geoffrey Rose presented the issue in his classic statement, risk factor research seeks the causes of cases, while population health seeks to understand the causes of the incidence rate. He observed that understanding why some individuals have hypertension is quite different from understanding why some populations have high rates and others low rates, and such questions require different types of studies and different approaches to interventions and social policy. The individual approach informs preventive efforts with high-risk individuals; the population health approach seeks to control the determinants of disease occurrence in large population groups.

The basic idea is easily understood, but, as Rose points out, some of the implications may not be obvious. Although persons at highest risk account for a disproportionate amount of illness, they are only a small minority of the population, and thus most cases of disease will occur among persons with little or moderate risk, because these populations are much more numerous. This means that simply focusing on high-risk individuals, in contrast to the entire population, will miss most disease and many of the cultural, normative, and environmental forces that shape disease patterns. Most people who have heart attacks and strokes have normal blood pressure; most people who suffer fractures have normal bone density; and so on. One implication is that we medicate everyone as in the polypill proposal noted earlier. An alternative is to seek population approaches that reduce disease incidence.

Another insight of the population health approach is that bringing about relatively small changes in average values in the population may result in big reductions in disease and mortality, but such measures do not offer any single individual much expected advantage in the short term. Rose refers to this as the "Prevention Paradox." People are far more motivated when they believe they personally are at risk and can substantially benefit from an intervention than when the risk is remote and the personal benefit of action is probabilistic and small. Policy makers similarly often have such views, willing to support heroic and expensive treatments after people have become ill much more enthusiastically than they support population and public health measures. The experience of September 11, the growth of terrorism, the threat of an avian flu epidemic, and the threat of biological, chemical, and nuclear attacks might make the importance of population health and public health more salient. The extent to which we have allowed our public health infrastructure to deteriorate is extremely dangerous.

Scientists who think in population health terms look to address broad influences that promote or threaten health. They are concerned with the built environment and the extent to which the organization of communities, housing, and transportation networks facilitate healthy living, allow for safe recreation, make it easy to obtain nutritious food and have a healthy diet, and protect children and the community from crime, dangerous traffic patterns, and noxious pollutants.[10] As travel is increasingly global, they seek to put into place systems to identify the spread of infectious disease and prevent epidemics. They seek to encourage healthy lifestyles not simply by exhorting individuals but by seeking to modify how work and play are organized and how routines in life naturally encourage people to live in a healthier way. They seek to prevent vehicle injuries and deaths as much by mandating safer vehicle design and improved highway systems as by driver education, licensing, and driver surveillance. They seek to get junk food out of schools, reduce TV watching, and involve children in group activities and community helping, and to build a sense of common purpose. They aspire to reduce exposure to tobacco and other harmful substances by regulating producers and distributors not only of noxious substances but also of unhealthy foods, soft drinks, and other unhealthy products that youngsters are drawn to.

Socioeconomic Status and Mortality

One of the most consistent observations in studies of disease and death is the large and persistent relationship between indicators of social class and poor health outcomes, with those at greatest social disadvantage having the highest death rates.[11] This relationship has been observed over more than a century in studies in Europe and North America; in more recent periods this relationship has been surprisingly large despite large improvements in overall living standards. Studies of earlier periods in European history suggest that the class relationship was not always present, indicating the importance of understanding why this relationship has been so large and persistent in recent times.[12]

Social class is a theoretical concept that seeks to characterize the hierarchical structuring of communities and societies and the way social groups relate to one another. The concept is conceived differently within varying theories of social stratification. Most contemporary empirical studies of mortality are tied less to broad social class theories and more to quantitative measures of socioeconomic status (SES). The most common measures used in empirical studies are income, education, occupation, and occupational rank. Studies of defined communities also sometimes use residence as a further indicator, and those using large data sets may characterize where the person lives as measured by the average income or education, racial composition, or average housing vales of particular geographic areas such as zip code areas or census tracts. Income, education, and occupational rank are highly associated, but each explains an independent portion of observed differences in mortality and morbidity when introduced individually in multivariate analyses.[13]

In American society, lower socioeconomic status is also highly correlated with being nonwhite and being Hispanic, although some ethnic groups, such as immigrants from some Asian countries, and their descendants, have higher incomes than the native white population.[14] Researchers believe that many of the racial differences in mortality and morbidity are due to socioeconomic factors, although some effects may be specific to race, such as the lower birth weights of black infants vis-à-vis white infants of comparable gestation and socioeconomic status, or outcomes linked to specific diseases associated with race such as sickle cell anemia or to the unique influences of racial discrimination. Many of these relationships such as birth weight are highly complex, since their determinants are intergenerational. The birth weight of a child, for example, depends on intrauterine conditions, which depend on the health status of the mother and her nutritional history, and thus the socioeconomic conditions of her upbringing. In any case, the white/nonwhite classification is commonly used as a proxy for SES when the data sets being used have no other SES information.

Understanding the role of social class and socioeconomic status as its proxy in explaining health and mortality is complex and challenging. Education, income, and occupation are associated with almost every aspect of life, including where and how people live, their food availability and nutrition, their exposure to environmental assaults such as pollution, traffic, and crime, risk of injury and death at the workplace, the extent of deprivation and stress in their lives, their sense of power and control over their lives, health knowledge and information, access to medical care, and diet, exercise, and many other important health related behaviors. These complex interconnections may operate differently for individual diseases and at different stages of the life course.[15] Environmental challenges such as environmental stressors or pollutants may interact differently with genetic and biological susceptibilities and at various stages of human development. For example, infants and children are more susceptible to damage from exposure to lead and other neurotoxins than adults are. Unraveling these complex causal networks is no small challenge. Many studies of SES and mortality are general analyses of overall trends, not refined analyses that allow sophisticated understanding of causal interrelationships.

Analysts think about SES relationships in several ways. The dominant epidemiological view is that SES is associated with various risk factors such as smoking, eating behavior, diet, exercise patterns, other substance use, and risk taking. Those following this line of thinking believe that identifying all the risk factors associated with SES that are also directly associated with mortality and other poor health outcomes will explain the real causes and suggest opportunities for intervention. Within this view, SES simply provides clues to the causes of mortality or disease or at best is an indirect cause through its influence on more proximate factors. This epidemiological perspective represents the viewpoint of most public health practitioners, who seek to identify and then intervene in order to change the presumed causal factors such as diet, lack of exercise, and high blood pressure.

Bruce Link and Jo Phelan have argued for an alternative view, one that sees SES as a fundamental cause of health and disease and not simply as a clue to more proximate factors.[16] Taking a historical perspective, they note that while risk factors change from one era to another as we ameliorate risks, the strong association between SES and health outcomes persists and may even get larger. Thus, they believe, there is something about SES that transcends any particular collection of risk factors. They argue that SES is fundamental in that persons of high status who have more power and influence and access to resources, information, and relationships have advantages in any era regardless of the existing specific risk factors, if human action makes it possible to prevent or ameliorate them. In short, higher-status people are more likely to know what they can do at any given time to prevent disease and death, and to have access to the instruments of prevention. In this instance remedial interventions would be to ensure that all people, regardless of socioeconomic status, have access to the information and resources necessary to take advantage of existing knowledge, technologies, and opportunities.

The inequalities at issue are of many kinds including disparities in income, education, access to information, and connection to social resources. Link and Phelan note that those who have these advantages will always have the potential of better health, because they can take remedial action sooner and more appropriately. Thus, Link and Phelan believe, it is as important to address these capacities as it is to focus on specific risk factors. This argument has much merit at the theoretical level. but, in a society such as ours, there are large impediments to redistributing income or modifying hierarchical structures. There is broad agreement, however, about such areas as educational opportunity, providing access to medical care, and building civic engagement.

Few would disagree that one's position in life has important impact on health and disease, and those who are most socially and economically disadvantaged have worse health, more disability, and higher mortality. It is understood that persons with poor health have greater difficulty in obtaining a higher level of education and earning a suitable income (what are seen as selection effects), but there is substantial evidence that whatever selection effects exist due to illness and disability, and they may under some circumstances be significant, the effects of poverty on health are large. An important observation, given much visibility through the Whitehall studies in the United Kingdom, is that the association between social standing and health outcomes is not only among the disadvantaged but continues up the SES scale.[17] The Whitehall studies showed, for example, that mortality decreased among English civil servants at each rung up the occupational hierarchy. Michael Marmot argues that since the civil servants in question were all employed workers with decent benefits, the findings suggest influences that go well beyond those typically associated with economic deprivation.

The Whitehall investigations are impressive, but it is wrong to assume that the different outcomes associated with occupational grade are simply a product of one's occupational standing. There may, in fact, be large selection biases, particularly at the higher rungs where those who achieve the highest positions are different from those below them in characteristics that are unmeasured but in some ways significantly health related. An important fact about the SES gradient is that the health effects are much larger among subgroups lower in the hierarchy than at higher levels. Most researchers accept the reality of the SES gradient in relation to health and mortality, but they significantly differ in how they interpret it.

Some believe that hierarchy itself, independent of income or education, has significance, because persons at higher positions have more autonomy and control over their work and their lives and because persons' location in the status hierarchy affect self-judgments and those of others and may lead some with lower status to a sense of relative deprivation.[18] Here advocates draw on work in health psychology and psychosocial epidemiology that has amassed much evidence on the relationships between psychological states and physiological responses.

A major stream of research in this vein examines the relationship between mortality patterns and income inequalities among developed nations, among states in the United States, and among provinces in Canada.[19] These broad analyses, dependent largely on ecological studies, have reported that inequalities in income, independent of the effects of income, are associated with disadvantageous mortality outcomes. There are significant methodological disputes concerning these data, and different studies using varying data sources, measures, and methods find disparate results. The findings in studies of mortality among nations are highly sensitive to the countries included in the analyses, and in some cases the observed results are dependent on very few data points. Studies of states, in contrast, may provide more convincing data, but investigators using different control variables get varied results.[20] Findings in studies in the United States tend to be confounded by different race and educational distributions among states, and each of these has been posited by some researchers as more important than income inequalities in understanding mortality.[21] The studies purporting to establish a relationship between income inequality and health have been reviewed extensively, and dissected, and a reasonable conclusion is that although there may be some effects in relation to particular causes of death (such as homicide), there is at best small empirical support for the influence of inequality independent of the effects of differences in income, education, and racial composition.

A number of interpretations have been suggested to account for the gradient noted in the Whitehall and other studies. One common explanation, consistent with many experimental investigations and other studies, attributes some of these findings to the individual's autonomy at work and control over the timing and pace of work. Certainly, persons in lower-ranking occupations, on average, have less discretion over timing and pace of work, are more closely supervised, and have less autonomy. Such factors have been associated with coronary risk and higher levels of distress. But these differences are unlikely to be large enough across the entire span of occupational levels to explain the gradient in mortality. Another explanatory approach draws from primate studies on hierarchies and dominance to argue that hierarchy itself, and being under the control of individuals with greater power and control, has negative health effects.[22] It is plausible that those with little power, and under the control of others, may experience adverse psychological and physical consequences, but again it seems far-fetched to believe that these influences can explain the gradient, particularly as persons ascend higher occupational rungs.

A third common interpretation is one of relative deprivation. Broad exposure through television, movies, and other media to people with affluent lifestyles and, as some have argued, awareness of the extraordinarily high compensation enjoyed by CEOs and other executives, elicits strong psychological feelings of relative deprivation that adversely affect physical and psychological functioning. Ironically, some of the posited health differences are empirically observed across large aggregations but have not been found within smaller geographic areas. The major proponent of this interpretation, Richard Wilkinson, has argued that one would expect the effects of relative deprivation to be seen primarily across large areas.[23] The difficulty with this view is that the large body of psychological research on relative deprivation finds that people typically compare themselves and how they are doing to others like themselves and not to celebrities, CEOs, or others distant in status. I compare myself to other researchers and professors, and not to the president of the United States, U.S. senators, or the heads of large corporations, or for that matter, even to lawyers, surgeons, or storekeepers.

In short, while the gradient is important for theoretical reasons, the fact that the effects of SES are much larger at lower levels in the occupational hierarchy suggests that this is where our interventions should be focused. Deprivations associated with poor schooling, poor housing, inferior diets, and polluted environments are more important than any differences between, for example, professional and higher executive grades, or between teachers and doctors. A number of points should be clear, however. Patterns of health and disease are the culmination of many factors. Thus, the story is likely to be very different depending on the causes of mortality, whether heart disease, cancer, homicide, or suicide. Any simple interpretation, however innovative and compelling, will not tell the whole story.

Although researchers aspire to explain causality, nonexperimental studies never completely eliminate selection effects. The selective forces in social life are very powerful, and, although luck is not irrelevant, where people end up in the occupational, educational, and income hierarchies is not a random process. Certainly, some part of the gradient is a result of selective factors, including differences in early socialization, motivation, cultural attitudes, and genetics. This remains a fruitful area for continuing inquiry. From a policy perspective, however, it would be wise to focus on the lower part of the SES distribution.

It should be noted that some believe that focusing on the gradient has social value because it suggests that we all share common causes of poor health and that awareness should therefore elicit more societal interest and concern. There is limited support for programs solely targeted to the poor, and much resistance to income redistribution and increased taxation. It is argued that if we all saw ourselves as being at risk and potentially benefiting from similar social interventions, we might be more supportive of large health and other social interventions. This may or may not be true, but the notion that inequality itself is a significant source of poor health has little empirical support. Ironically, while inequality in the United States, the United Kingdom, and in much of the world has increased, the trajectory of longevity in these and most other nations continues in a favorable direction.

Racial and Ethnic Disparities

The size and importance of racial disparities have been documented repeatedly in many studies and reviews.[24] In the United States, African Americans, Native Americans, and selected Hispanic populations, especially Mexican Americans, face the largest disparities in insurance coverage, access to care, and appropriate treatment. African Americans and Native Americans face the highest burdens of mortality and morbidity compared with the U.S. white population.[25] Some of these disparities are explained by differences in education and income, but even at comparable levels of SES, disparities persist as a result of many factors, including racial discrimination, geographic concentration in high-poverty environments with undeveloped or depleted infrastructures, cultural orientations of patients and providers, and language problems. It is stated U.S. government policy to eliminate disparities in health, and access to health resources, but programmatic efforts do not match the rhetoric.

While we speak in overall summary terms about these issues and thus avoid messy complexity, such discussions tend to be misleading. There is much variation affecting every aspect of the issue: group classifications, whether African American, Hispanic, Asian, or any other, include much heterogeneity; the outcomes being evaluated range from insurance coverage to mortality; the characteristics of populations even within a given category differ in terms of language, culture, geography, education, acculturation, and social networks. As noted earlier, some ethnic groups do better than the native-born white population; many do worse. There are significant differences between Spanish-speaking populations from Cuba and Chile and those from Puerto Rico and Mexico. And in each case, those from educated backgrounds are very different from those with little education. Many immigrant groups from Taiwan, India, and elsewhere come with higher education and many skills, enter white-collar jobs, and do comparatively well;[26] others come from situations of great disadvantage and chaotic circumstances and experience a hard time. Social selection again is an important factor, since those who seek to emigrate are different in important ways from the populations they leave behind. The composition of immigrant groups from a country may change from one period to another, as, for example, the pre-1980 Cuban immigration after the Castro revolution compared with the Cubans boat-lifted from the Port of Mariel.[27]

Much of the work on disparities mixes good analysis with advocacy and political correctness, which can get in the way of thoughtful policy discussion. We need quite different remedies for varying subgroups, and it is important not to overgeneralize. For many immigrant groups, and some Hispanic populations, language difficulties are a major barrier to obtaining appropriate care, but the problems for African Americans are quite different. Much of the research on disparities is focused on the African American population and its high levels of infant and adult mortality and morbidity. But even here, it is important to differentiate between those born here, immigrants from various African nations and those from the Caribbean, with their different social histories and predispositions.[28] Although all these groups face racial discrimination because of dominant stereotypes, even such stereotypes and discrimination may be more differentiated than we usually assume. Understanding and doing something tangible about disparities requires a specific focus on each evident barrier.

Many of the race and ethnic inequalities that are of concern are not simply a matter of racism and discrimination, although these obviously exist, but even more products of multiple factors that come together to produce their effects. Understanding the relatively low health insurance coverage of Mexican Americans, for example, requires understanding not only their poverty and ethnicity but also their geographic residence, the types of jobs they have, the fact that many of their employers, dominant in agriculture, do not provide health insurance coverage and the like. There is an extensive literature showing that black patients with particular diagnoses do not receive comparable cutting-edge care that white patients receive. This is not only generally the case but also very true of Medicare, where everyone theoretically has comparable coverage. Explanations vary from prejudice and discrimination to differences in attitudes, illness behavior, and effective communication with physicians. But often people with the same coverage cannot cash it in equally because of lack of access due to where they live and what providers are available to them. A recent study found, for example, that black Medicare patients receive poorer quality of care than white patients because they are treated by different primary care physicians who on average are less well trained and less adequately positioned to get them access to high-quality specialists and technical services.[29]

Policy makers who aspire to eliminate barriers to access appropriate services and better health commonly assume that promoting population health and reducing disparities are two sides of the same coin. Major initiatives to improve population health, which may substantially improve the health of disadvantaged groups among others, may in fact counterintuitively increase rather than diminish disparities. Policy makers sometimes may have to decide which objective should receive highest priority. Some believe that the existence of disparities is inconsistent with a fair society and favor initiatives to reduce disparities even if an alternative investment could produce better health for all, including the health of minorities, but at the cost of enlarging disparities. Others would argue, as I would, that the most important goal is improving the health of all groups and that we should seek to get the most health possible out of our investments. An examination of infant mortality makes the distinction clear.[30]

Black infant mortality has been approximately one and a half times to double the white infant mortality rate for decades, although both blacks and whites have benefited from advances in living conditions and medical technologies that have significantly reduced infant mortality. In 1950, nonwhite infant mortality was 43.9 deaths per thousand live births, 64 percent higher than the white rate of 26.8. Over the next forty-eight years, nonwhite infant mortality fell to 13.8 deaths per thousand live births compared to 6 for whites, a disparity about twice as large as before. However, in every five-year period since 1965, more nonwhite than white lives were saved per one thousand live births. Over the entire period since 1950, 50 percent more nonwhite babies per thousand born were saved than white babies. Everyone gained with advances in living conditions and medical technology, and more black than white lives were saved, but the disparity ratio increased substantially. An important issue is whether for policy purposes it makes more sense to focus on calculations of lives saved than on disparity ratios per se.

There are two explanations for the relationship between health improvements and disparity ratios. One is a relatively trivial statistical fact that as we get to small numbers, small differences in cases can yield large differences in ratios. Yet any sensible person understands that while the differences between five and ten and between five hundred and one thousand yield the same ratio, these numbers may have very different significance. More importantly, health initiatives that depend to some degree on voluntary participation and cooperation will inevitably favor those who are more advantaged in access and resources, another implication of the Link-Phelan conception of SES as a fundamental cause. If given access to information and resources, disadvantaged groups will eventually reach the levels attained by the more advantaged in any area of modifiable health outcomes, but the gap can persist for long time periods. Targeted programs focused on those at greatest risk can help close the gap more quickly, but inevitably those with more resources will have a lead as the next new opportunity arises.

Another implication of the concept of fundamental cause is that, to the extent that preventive and promotive health efforts are involuntary and outside the decisions and motivations of each individual, disparities are less likely to occur. Thus, fluoridation of water is less likely to result in disparities in tooth decay than dependence on instruction in teeth brushing; air bags are less likely to lead to disparities than seat belts; and fortified food is more likely to eliminate disparities than teaching people about healthy diets. Similarly, ensuring that the entire population has health insurance and that needed care is geographically and socially accessible is far more effective than expecting people to work these things out on their own. Disparities in health outcomes are also more likely to occur in disease areas where preventive opportunities are abundant than those where we know little about prevention. Thus, we have large disparities among groups in lung cancer but much smaller ones in cancer of the pancreas. This point about preventability may help explain why in earlier periods in European history the social class gradient was not evident, given how little knowledge there was about what could be prevented and how.

Population Health and Culture Change

Public health has always had more political difficulty than curative medicine because its initiatives often come into conflict with social and political ideologies and economic interests, including those of curative medicine itself. Population health endeavors face many of the same conflicts. It may be self evident to the public health practitioner that health is promoted by sex education in the schools and the availability of contraception, that lives can be saved by giving clean needles to IV drug users who are at risk of AIDS, that many, including children, die unnecessarily because of poor control over guns and their availability, and that the promotion of high-calorie foods and drinks to children contributes to obesity and future chronic disease. But in each case strong religious, ideological, and economic forces frame these issues differently and believe their values and interests should trump any public health interest.

In contrast to issues that stir political and ideological emotions, there are many others around which there is more consensus about many potentially valuable interventions; these include efforts to reduce the incidence of cancer and heart disease, address the growing problem of obesity, promote child health, and protect the public from contaminants proven to be toxic. Most people enthusiastically endorse these goals and support reasonable initiatives to address them. But many of the changes we aspire to at the community level require changing how people go about their daily lives—that is, norms and culture—and this is a much tougher challenge. There have been successes, such as dramatic changes in how most of the public views smoking and the norms that affect smoking behavior, but even this has been a long and difficult endeavor that requires continuing renewal.

Initiatives to reduce smoking have been introduced in many ways, including public education, individual smoking-cessation treatment, increased taxation of cigarettes, limiting minors' access to cigarettes, restrictions on advertising, and litigation. But the changing public views of smoking and the restrictions that were made possible as social norms changed probably had as much influence as any other factor in reducing smoking among the American population. While in the past it was viewed as impolite, and even highly eccentric, to ask people not to smoke at meetings, in the workplace, and even in one's home, changing norms put smokers on the defensive. The increased restrictions on smoking in public places such as restaurants, airports, public buildings, transport, and even in bars put smokers on the defensive and contributed to devaluing and stigmatizing their behavior. Some employers penalize or even fire workers for smoking at home, leading to plausible protests about a nanny state. This massive culture change in the United States becomes more evident as one travels around the world where the older cigarette culture continues to prevail. No doubt the evidence of the dangers of secondhand smoke played a significant part as the case was made to the public that smokers were endangering others' health as well as their own. The antismoking campaign had many advantages: unequivocal documentation of smoking's large and harmful consequences; strong support from governmental health agencies and their leaders; documentation of a history of lying and deceptions by the tobacco industry; effective public advocacy and litigation approaches;[31] and evidence that secondhand smoke harmed children and others in the smoker's household. Despite all this, the battle against tobacco is far from won. There have been other population health victories, although not without long battles, for example, removing from paints and gasoline the lead that has harmed the brain development of children.[32] However tough it has been to overcome the views of smokers and the interests of industries that manufacture harmful substances, these may be relatively easy challenges compared to future endeavors related to unhealthy foods, guns, SUVs, and much more.

In recent years considerable discussion has focused on social capital and the building of civic communities, an idea popularized by Putnam and others.[33] Social capital, in contrast to the human capital often discussed by economists, speaks to the resources that people draw from their connections to others in the web of social relationships. Putnam focuses on the positive aspects of social ties and social and political participation and the access it gives for practical help, social support, information, and access to people and opportunities. But social ties also have a darker side and can restrict behavior and affect outcomes in negative ways. Much depends on the values and norms of the individual networks and the influences they have. Belonging to a street gang may provide as much social capital as belonging to a civic group that serves the community, but the former case may encourage substance use, crime, and violence. Strong social and religious ties, in some contexts, may discourage advanced schooling, leaving the household and neighborhood, and exercising one's preferences and opinions. The difficulty in some Muslim societies that discourage female education is not that they lack social capital but that they encourage attitudes and behavior that limit women's participation in community activities and educational and civic affairs. Female education is an excellent predictor of the survival of women's future children.[34] In short, the value context is all important. There is a world of difference between connectedness to a neo-Nazi subculture or a terrorist group, where ties may be extremely strong, and the Salvation Army or the League of Women Voters, and the latter are different from participation in bowling leagues and sports teams.

If one considers health behavior specifically, the same observations apply. Strong social networks, group cohesiveness, and trust may enable the group to influence behavior, but the content of behavior depends on whether the group values preventive health action, scientific medicine, and active engagement with illness when it occurs.[35] These predispositions may be embedded deeply in the group's culture and religious and social ideologies. The good health of Mormons results not only from prohibitions on smoking, drinking, and recreational sexual activity but also from promotion of a quiet and stable life with strong kinship loyalties, attention to childhood socialization, a positive orientation to education, and a strong emphasis on the work ethic. Mormonism does more than prohibit substances; it teaches the importance of family relationships and parenthood and encourages mastery of the environment, effort, and accomplishment.[36] But there are many ways to live, and some prefer the excitement of Las Vegas to Salt Lake City. Comparison of these two cities indicates that while they face many similar environmental circumstances, their cultures produce different levels of health,[37] but the rub is that not everyone wants to live like Mormons.

In short, building population health is no simple matter and is not open to quick fixes. It is a component of a larger culture war, caught in the battles between the Puritan ethic and the social gospel as Morone has described it in his history of how morality affects health.[38] Population health efforts must be attentive to the character of a free society, the strong individualistic orientations of persons and groups, and the fact that while everyone wants good health, health is not the ultimate value that trumps all others. Population health advocates must look for opportunities where the cultural consensus supports them or act on new opportunities as they emerge. The overall mission must be multifaceted, working at many levels, from individual to community to social policy.

Chapter 4

The Murky Challenge of Mental Health

The term "mental health" is one almost everyone uses, but it has no clear or consistent meaning. The mental health specialty sector commonly refers to its domain as behavioral health, covering the provision of services for psychiatric disorders and substance abuse problems. Behavioral factors affect almost every aspect of health and health care, including the occurrence of health problems, people's conceptions of sickness and what is wrong, decisions to seek help, cooperation and response to treatment, and the course and chronicity of illness. Mental health, broadly defined, is important to all aspects of medicine and medical care. Mental health is also a specialized sector of the health care system, diagnosing and treating people with psychiatric disorders. It is estimated that in 2001, $104 billion dollars was spent specifically on mental health and substance abuse treatment, making up 7.6 percent of all health care expenditures for that year.[1] Most of the total, $85 billion went for mental health services and $18 billion for treatment for substance abuse.

Mental health problems are of great importance and major causes of distress, disability, and even death. Nevertheless, mental illness remains a murky and confusing area. The number of diagnoses increase in each version of the *Diagnostic and Statistical Manual of Mental Disorders* (DSM), the bible for psychiatric diagnosis, from 106 in *DSM-I* in 1952 to 297 in the 1994 version, *DSM-IV*.[2] Although there are many real mental disorders of vital importance to health, others are dicey and strongly contested, reflecting committee votes based on little science. Perhaps the most extreme case was the removal of homosexuality from the *DSM* in 1973 by vote, accompanied by lobbying and demonstrations.

Treatments for many patients with comparable conditions are provided by psychiatrists, psychologists, general physicians, social workers, counselors, nurses, clergy, complementary and alternative practitioners, and still others, including consumer services and self-help groups. Of those said to have a mental illness who were studied between 2001and 2003, only two-fifths had had care from anyone in the prior year, and fewer received treatment from a psychiatrist than from a complementary and alternative therapist.[3] Mental health is a bit of a topsy-turvy world, with many more persons with serious mental illness in jails and prisons than in psychiatric hospitals, and some of the most seriously ill and impaired patients are on the streets, commonly homeless, with little care at all.

Historically, mental health and mental health treatment have been separate from the main provision of medical care and were mostly a state government responsibility. Mental health care was largely provided in isolated asylums, separate from other medical institutions, and care was primarily for persons we would today view as the most seriously and persistently mentally ill.[4] Patterns of mental health care have changed dramatically as the range of treated conditions has expanded greatly, the number deemed in need of mental health treatment has increased enormously, new treatments have become available, and a large range of professionals in addition to psychiatrists provide mental health services.[5]

Public resources accounted for 63 percent of 2001 expenditures, and public payments remain a more important source of mental health coverage than they are for general medical services. States and localities continue to play a dominant role through Medicaid (accounting for 44 percent of public mental health and substance abuse treatment expenditures) and other state and local disbursements (accounting for 37 percent). The direct federal role in mental health is more limited; Medicare and other federal funds account for only about one-fifth of all public mental health expenditures. Unlike earlier periods, when most expenditures supported state and county custodial mental hospitals, the largest expenditures now go for outpatient care, retail drugs, inpatient care in general hospitals, and residential care. In the ten years between 1991 and 2001, almost two-fifths of the growth in expenditures was for medications, which now are the single biggest cost for mental health in state Medicaid programs.

The numbers of clients treated, or those said to be in need, or the increased numbers of providers of these services alone do not convey why mental health is so important to the health of the population. Doctors have long recognized that many patients who seek assistance, reporting common and ubiquitous physical complaints, seem motivated as much by psychological distress and difficult and seemingly intractable problems in their lives as by the specific physical complaints they present to the doctor.[6] These days, in the United States, these patients are typically characterized as depressed and anxious, or as somatizing patients, and by clinicians less sympathetic as "worried wells" or, sometimes, hypochondriacs. In an earlier time, and still in some regions in the world, such patients were seen as having neurasthenia, often regarded as a neurological nervous condition, or as being neurotic.[7] However such patients were perceived and defined, clinicians recognized that they consulted frequently, complained chronically, amplified common physical problems, and were difficult to reassure. They also found that such patients often had other illnesses exacerbated by their distress, and that these distressed psychological states contributed to decrements in performing usual roles, including meeting work and family responsibilities. Subsequently, many studies documented these patterns,[8] but this too fails to convey the importance of mental health and well-being to the health of the population.

In this chapter I focus primarily on the treatment of psychiatric disorders and the specialty mental health sector. But fully appreciating the broad role of mental health requires an examination of how people think about their health and well-being, and what they commonly mean when they indicate that their health is poor.

Public Conceptions of Health

It is common in medicine to define health as the absence of known disease, since this is more easily definable and measurable than positive states of well-being. But if researchers ask people to assess their own health and then examine the predictors of such ratings, they invariably find such assessments to have several dimensions. First, as one would assume, the existence and severity of acute physical and chronic health problems are associated with ratings of poorer health. Invariably, depression and other types of distress contribute to poor ratings of overall health as well. And, perhaps surprisingly, life problems in a social sense and psychosocial stress, what some call social health, sometimes contribute to these self-assessments. Fundamentally, people view their health in broad terms, in terms of present or impending threats to fulfilling their usual life responsibilities, and in relation to their capacity to engage fully in valued activities.[9]

It might be argued that medicine is an applied science and that people's definitions and feelings about their health have limited relevance to building evidence-based practice and capitalizing on scientific advancements. What really counts, one might say, are objective findings about what prevents, ameliorates, or cures disease, limits disabilities, and lengthens life. Interventions, however, depend on people's cooperation in using the health system and in their treatment; without their cooperation achievements are limited. Even more telling is the fact that people's assessments of their health predict future outcomes and death more successfully than physician assessments or risk-factor measurement.[10] This predictive ability is not well understood, but people seem able to perceive aspects of their health that expert judgments and scientific tests do not capture. Many longitudinal studies carried out with populations in a variety of nations find that self-assessments of health successfully predict outcomes even decades in advance, controlling for known risk factors associated with morbidity and mortality. This, and much other work, makes clear that the psychosocial dimensions of health and medical care transcend the treatment and care typically carried out in the mental health sector.

This should not be surprising, since the body and mind are one. We speak about mental and physical events in dualistic language, but they are two sides of the same coin. The brain is a physical organ, and while we have yet to understand consciousness, all psychological states are embodied in our physiology. Communication, whether in psychotherapeutic endeavors, in ordinary doctor patient interactions, in relationships with significant others and loved ones, or even in other social relationships, can have powerful effects on perceptions, emotions, and bodily reactions that have important impact on well-being. It is well established that the placebo effect in medical care is a powerful influence, making it necessary to evaluate drugs and treatments through randomized controlled studies that assess the efficacy of treatment beyond effects of suggestibility (the placebo effect). Good medical care is as much about empathy, communication, and persuasion as it is about tests, drugs, and procedures. But all aspects of behavior or mental health cannot realistically or practically be the object of medical attention. Much inevitably must remain within the province of the usual problems of living and the many struggles people have in coping with life problems, fulfilling their hopes and aspirations, and dealing with disappointments.

Psychiatric Disorder, Patterns of Help-Seeking, and the Role of the Mental Health Specialty Sector

Epidemiological studies of the U.S. population estimate that in any given year between one-quarter and one-third of the population have sufficient symptoms to meet criteria for a mental illness as defined by *DSM-IV*,[11] the diagnostic and statistical manual for clinicians developed by committees of the American Psychiatric Association. These community surveys further find that approximately one-half the population have had such disorders at some point in their lives. Many people agree that the DSM categories and their criteria are overinclusive and that many persons said to have disorders would not want or need treatment, nor would they necessarily benefit from treatment.[12] These large estimates at first impress the public as astonishing because the public's image of mental illness, based on acute psychotic disorders such as schizophrenia or bipolar disease commonly depicted in the media, is quite different from most of the conditions these surveys measure. If one makes the analogy with so-called physical illness, remember that most people, most of the time, have symptoms that could be classified as an illness based on the *International Classification of Disease*, but most of these conditions are not harmful and many are self-limited and do not require medical intervention. Thus, it is less important to know that many people can be given a diagnosis, and more important to know how serious their conditions are, the extent to which they are disabling or interfere with life functions and satisfactions, and whether they would improve with treatment. As with physical illness, the National Comorbidity Study (NCS) found that while conditions were common, serious illness commonly involving additional psychiatric conditions (comorbidity) was much more limited. Many people who are said to have mental illnesses in these surveys do not seek or want treatment, or prefer to handle their distress on their own. Whether such persons are correct in such judgments or respond this way because of stigma, lack of knowledge about how they could be helped, or other barriers, remains an issue.

Researchers recognize that having an illness is not the same as having a need for treatment, and they make various efforts to distinguish need by linking disorders with further information on the extent to which the disorder interferes with everyday life and leads to difficulties in functioning in usual family, work, and community roles.[13] Such linkage reduces the estimates of the number of people said to be mentally ill, but they remain quite large. Experts disagree about whether the adjustments used in these revised definitions are scientifically meaningful or are simply arbitrary corrections to make the numbers appear more credible.[14] Moreover, even among this more delimited population, most persons defined as having a mental illness neither perceive a need nor seek care.

Efforts are further made to identify the subpopulation within this larger group who can be said to have serious and persistent mental illnesses.[15] These estimates take into account comorbid conditions, the extent of disability associated with psychiatric conditions, and the duration of the disorder. Conditions typically seen as serious include schizophrenia, affective psychoses, bipolar disease, major depression, panic disorder, and obsessive-compulsive disorders, but these diagnoses are quite heterogeneous and include persons with varying needs. Some persons having diagnoses that are believed to be less serious may as a consequence have high levels of disability and have serious needs. Thus, diagnoses by themselves are not determinative. Many mental illnesses, like many respiratory diseases, get better on their own after a short period of time. Estimates of the severe subgroup tend to be in the 5 to 10 percent range in contrast to the commonly cited one-third to one-half, but in a population approaching 300 million people, the number of people requiring serious attention is still very large, in the vicinity of 15 to 30 million people. If one focuses on the most impaired persons, those who require intensive and continuing care, it probably is more in the 2 to 3 percent range.

Most people who have mental illnesses with persistent disabling symptoms eventually seek and receive some mental health care, although sometimes after years of delay.[16] Mental health professionals advocate early interventions, but intervening early in the case of less serious disorders inevitably provides care to many persons who will get better by themselves. Psychiatry is not very proficient at differentiating self-limited disorders, such as those associated with transitory life stresses, from others that will become more chronic.

In some countries where psychiatry and other mental health clinicians function primarily as part of a referral consultant service, the specialized mental health sector primarily treats those with the most severe and persistent illnesses. The situation is more complicated in the United States, because patients positively inclined toward psychiatry and psychotherapy often come directly to the specialty sector. Thus, who is treated at different locations and by varying practitioners depends in part on the way people seek care, their attitudes about different types of practitioners, and their insurance coverage. In the National Comorbidity Study, repeated a second time (NCS-R), one-third of all mental health visits were made by persons with no apparent disorders.[17] Although such persons are much less likely to use care than those who meet clinical criteria for the many conditions studied, they are a large part of the population and use much of available resources. While some patients seek assistance directly from psychiatrists, psychologists, and mental health centers and clinics, others will accept services from their primary care doctor but resist being diagnosed as having a psychiatric illness and being referred to the specialty sector. Those who are treated in the specialty sector are often there by virtue of their own treatment decisions, because they are willing to accept specialty referral, and because their primary care doctor is willing to refer them in situations when a referral is required. Others come into psychiatric services because of family pressures or because public authorities intervene when their behavior becomes disruptive.

The Role of the Specialty Mental Health Sector

The networks of help-seeking and provision of mental health services are untidier in the United States than in many other countries because of the proliferation of varying types of practitioners offering behavioral services and the preferences and care-seeking inclinations of patients. Care provision does not follow any clear, rational plan; nevertheless, important policy decisions are needed about which mental health services should be covered by health insurance, the criteria that should govern eligibility for receiving insured services, and the special role of psychiatry and the larger specialized mental health sector relative to other treatment providers such as primary care physicians, who provide one-third to one-half of all treatment, depending upon how it is defined. Historically, mental health insurance coverage has been more limited than coverage for treatment for most medical conditions, and mental health advocates have been committed to achieving insurance parity, that is, providing mental illness insurance on the same basis as for other medical conditions. Many states have passed legislation insuring some parity in coverage, and there have been legislation and other parity requirements at the federal level as well, as in the Federal Employee's Health Benefits (FEHB) program, but full parity remains an unfulfilled goal. Parity does not ensure access or increased quality. A major study of introducing parity in the FEHB program found only very modest changes in access to care, utilization, costs, or quality.[18] In most plans studied, clients had fewer out-of-pocket costs as a result of parity, however.

A major controversy underlying the parity issue, and discussions of mental health insurance issues more generally, involves the definition of what mental health problems should be seen as medically relevant and which are better characterized as adjustment problems, problems in coping with common life stresses, and more ordinary problems of living. These may seem like artificial distinctions, but they are relevant in judging which problems should remain primarily the responsibility of individuals, their families, and informal networks and which should be covered by insurance as medical problems. In our consumer-oriented society, many believe that the need for services should remain self-defined, and those wishing treatment should be free to seek whatever help they believe they need. The right of people to purchase whatever services they want is not contested, but neither government nor private payers are willing, or should be required, to finance such an open-ended definition of care. This is especially true of psychotherapy, which many seek to achieve better self-understanding and self-actualization, and not necessarily for treating disorders.

Consider the case of psychoanalysis, a highly coveted and expensive form of psychotherapy, favored among some segments of the population in earlier decades. Psychoanalysis largely has been discredited as a form of medical treatment, but some still value it as a helpful form of self-inquiry. It is rare for insurance to pay for psychoanalysis any longer, and types of psychotherapy such as cognitive therapy and interpersonal therapy that are covered by insurance are more directive and time limited. The issue of insurance coverage for psychoanalysis raises the two types of key decisions that must be resolved more generally: how to define who should be eligible to receive services and what specific services should be paid for.

Some mental health advocacy groups, such as the influential National Alliance for the Mentally Ill (NAMI), argue for mental health insurance parity with physical coverage, but only for persons who are said to be seriously mentally ill, or in NAMI's terms, persons with disorders of the brain. The difficulty is that there is no clear way of distinguishing mental illnesses that are brain conditions from others. Thus, coverage comes to be based on an arbitrary listing of what are believed to be the most serious mental disorders, such as affective psychoses, schizophrenia, bipolar disorder, and major depression. The difficulty is that while such distinctions have a general plausibility as measures of need, there is no absolute relationship between diagnosis and impairments. Moreover, diagnostic distinctions do not take the effectiveness of available treatments into account.

In addition to eligibility and coverage, it is also necessary to determine the types of services to be provided and for how long, and which of the many types of clinicians and practitioners should be eligible to receive reimbursement for providing these services. Allowing additional types of clinicians to receive insurance reimbursement increases the provision of services and costs, and thus many types of mental health practitioners are excluded from receiving insurance reimbursement as a way of limiting costs. In addition, in the last decade or so, there has been a significant shift from traditional cost-constraint approaches to dependence on managed mental health care. The traditional approach provided only modest mental health coverage; it also limited care for covered services by means of high deductibles and high co-insurance (typically 50 percent for outpatient services compared with the usual 20 percent for physical illness), limits on the number of visits, and yearly and lifetime dollar limits. High cost sharing inhibited the use of outpatient care. In the case of inpatient care, the idea of being hospitalized on a psychiatric unit was in itself a sufficient inhibition, but inpatient care in any case was typically restricted to fifteen to forty-five days. A significant problem, was that, once hospitalized, patients were often kept in the hospital until their inpatient coverage was exhausted, a pattern of care viewed by policy makers as inefficient and wasteful. Average inpatient stays in psychiatry far exceeded those for most other conditions, and the reasons appeared to be more economic than medical.

The provision of mental health services changed substantially with the introduction of managed behavioral health care. Typically, Medicaid, insurance plans, and HMOs contract with managed behavioral health care organizations to administer the mental health part of insurance coverage, referred to as a mental health carve-out. Carve-outs take some piece of the overall insurance plan, such as mental health services, substance abuse services, child services, AIDS care, or medication management, and administer and manage them separately. This may be done on a risk basis, where the contracting organization receives a capitation for providing necessary services (a fixed amount for each covered enrollee), or on an administrative basis, receiving a fee for managing the benefit. The organization is then responsible for organizing a network of services, assessing patients and determining need, developing treatment plans, and monitoring the process of care. The managed care organization has more discretion than was characteristic of traditional care defined by specific insurance coverage, and it decides what care to provide, the extent to which less expensive professionals such as social workers substitute for more expensive psychiatrists, and the duration of treatment. Traditional patient cost-sharing arrangements no longer apply, making services more accessible to the patient from a cost perspective. Economists refer to this as substituting restraints on the supply side for traditional restraints on the demand side.

Once patients enter the mental health specialty system, their care is managed through a range of utilization-control strategies. Managed care has increased initial access to specialty mental health care, but it has substantially reduced the intensity of care, particularly the use of extended inpatient care and long-term psychotherapy. In essence, managed care makes it easy for patient need to be assessed and for people to receive some mental health care, but it controls the services provided and the cost of those services. Most patients receive medication therapy and/or psychotherapy or counseling for a limited number of sessions. Managed care has substantially reduced the costs of mental health care with no indication that, for the population as a whole, care is any less effective than it was under the traditional but more costly fee-for-service system. Economies are achieved by avoiding much inpatient care, reducing the length of psychotherapy, using drug formularies, depending on less expensive clinicians than psychiatrists, and bargaining down reimbursement rates.[19]

The picture is more murky in the case of patients with serious and persistent conditions. The quality of care for these high-need patients varies depending on their health insurance plan and managed care arrangements, with some plans performing well and others poorly.[20] Relatively few patients in either traditional fee-for-service or managed care receive treatment consistent with evidence-based treatment norms for either schizophrenia or depression.[21] There is some evidence in managed care of services being distributed more equally among all patients treated than in fee-for-service care, leaving those most seriously ill with less intensive services than they may require.[22] There have also been problems in providing suitable mental health services for children, although it is not clear that the situation is any worse than in the traditional system.

Over time, the availability of traditional clinicians such as psychiatrists and psychiatric nurses has not expanded very much, but the supply of other mental health clinicians, such as social workers, counselors, and rehabilitation therapists, has substantially grown. Psychiatrists now primarily manage the medical aspects of treatment, such as medication and inpatient care, while most outpatient therapy is provided by other mental health professionals.[23] This is less expensive and is consistent with the growth of mental health services in a context of a limited supply of psychiatrists, but some experts worry about these now typical providers' lack of medical sophistication. Increasingly nurse practitioners, and now in some states physician assistants and psychologists, have been given legal authority to prescribe some psychiatric medications, and this trend may grow, particularly in geographic locations with few psychiatrists.

In the last decade or so the balance in mental health treatment has shifted toward much greater use of medications and less psychotherapy, in part because of the way care is now managed. About half of all mental health services is still provided outside the mental health specialty sector, largely by primary care physicians who mostly treat with medications and modest counseling. Such care, provided in primary care, typically fails to meet appropriate practice guidelines.[24] When patients enter the managed care specialty sector, many of the services are provided by nonphysicians, such as psychologists and social workers, but studies show that despite the untidiness of the overall sorting process, those with the most severe and persistent problems are most likely to end up under some psychiatric supervision.

New drugs, such as the selective serotonin reuptake inhibitors (SSRIs) for the treatment of depression and other psychiatric problems and the new atypical antipsychotic medications, are believed to have less disturbing side effects. Patients appear to tolerate them better, and general physicians with little mental health training are more comfortable with prescribing SSRIs than they were with earlier antidepressants. The pharmaceutical companies market these drugs aggressively to doctors, and to patients through direct-to-consumer advertising, and the increase in use has been phenomenal.[25] Ironically, there is no evidence that these drugs are any more effective than earlier ones, and they may even be less effective, although they are more acceptable to doctors and patients. Some evidence and experience suggest that the combination of medication and counseling (as in cognitive psychotherapy or interpersonal therapy) is superior to either alone in depression treatment,[26] but most patients who receive mental health care receive primarily drug treatment. Such treatment is less expensive and is believed to be quicker in relieving symptoms than psychotherapy, although it is not clearly superior overall in treating depression. In fact, some question whether these SSRIs are much superior to placebo and remain unconvinced of the studies that report their clinical utility.[27] From a practical standpoint it is important that new medications make it easier for doctors to treat depression and make less demand on the doctors' time and schedule, when typically doctors feel quite rushed.

Fit Between Need, Demand, and
the Use of Mental Health Services

Three types of mental health need and care have been defined. The first represents the many people who face troubles in their lives, feel miserable, and come to doctors seeking help, or present physical complaints that are amplified and made salient by their troubles. A second level includes those with disorders of mild or moderate severity, and those with a persistent disorder who are functioning in a stable way. These people need attention but the care they require is not intensive or expensive to provide. A third level involving patients with serious and persistent disorders, often combined with substance abuse and other psychiatric problems, and causing significant disability, are a critical group of patients needing much clinical and public policy attention.

Primary care clinicians are expected to provide caring and social support, to intervene with therapies to reduce depression and anxiety, and provide whatever tangible help is possible. They are also expected to refer more seriously disordered patients to mental health specialists and, not unimportantly, to avoid a medical trajectory that subjects these patients to countless diagnostic tests and other interventions that might reinforce self-defined illness, incur high costs unnecessarily, or even harm them. Finding the proper balance is more easily said than done, since physicians feel under pressure not to fail to recognize an undetected physical illness and some patients, unwilling to confront the idea that they have a psychiatric problem, not infrequently insist on more medical investigations. Some of this can be averted through careful listening and good communication, but primary care doctors work under much time pressure that makes it difficult to allocate the needed time. It is easier to send the patient for another procedure or test, particularly when patients are insistent, and often further investigations are remunerative for the medical organization as well.

There is abundant evidence that physicians often fail to recognize depression and other states of distress in their patients.[28] Good disease management programs and well-organized efforts to work with physician practices can substantially improve the recognition and care of depression,[29] the most common manifestation of psychological distress in primary care populations. Perhaps the single most important influence encouraging treatment of depression by primary care physicians has been the ease of using SSRIs, but these drugs commonly are not being provided in an appropriately evidence-based way. Persons treated in the mental health specialty sector are more likely to receive care that meets evidence-based standards than those treated in primary care.[30] SSRIs also have often been oversold; their effectiveness in treating patents with milder and more moderate symptoms is unproven. There is also concern that the use of some SSRIs with children and adolescents, and even possibly some adults, may occasionally increase an inclination to suicide, but the evidence remains uncertain.[31] Many experts believe that if primary care physicians devoted more time and attention to effective communication with troubled patients and those whose chronic disease is compounded by depression and anxiety,[32] some expensive and unnecessary interventions could be avoided. They also believe that patients given SSRIs and other psychiatric medications should be monitored carefully.

A second level of care includes those who have an acute mental disorder of mild or moderate severity, and continuing management of persons who have a chronic disorder but who are functioning in a stable way. These patients, as noted earlier, might be managed either by the primary care doctor, by an office-based mental health clinician, or by a mental health service that is part of a managed behavioral health carve-out. Here the challenge is to provide evidence-based treatment, monitor the patient, provide social support, and make referrals for other types of assistance that might be needed. Often the separation of needed services, as occurs in carve-outs, makes it difficult to coordinate care in meaningful ways. Various models of integrating medical and mental health services have been advocated, but the only approach that seems to work reasonably is close collaboration between consulting mental health professionals and primary care practitioners who take on the management of clients with mental illness.[33] Simply making a psychiatrist available as a consultant doesn't appear to help a great deal.

A third major subgroup of patients, and the most critical group from the perspective of social policy, is the group with severe and persistent problems. These were the patients who were traditionally put in mental hospitals, which provided many services, including housing, nutrition, activities, and medical care. Care in community settings, where many services that clients need are scattered geographically and among agencies, poses difficult challenges. Many patients do well and live satisfactory lives. Others, however, face difficult obstacles in getting the services they need and maintaining a decent quality of life.

People with mental illness who are seriously ill and impaired are typically managed in the specialty sector. Many are poor and depend on the Medicaid program for their care, which has become the single most important program for persons with serious mental illness and an indispensable safety net. Most states now depend on contracts with managed behavioral health care organizations to provide much of this care, and they have greatly reduced their roles as direct providers of service. While there are some excellent mental health Medicaid programs, care varies a great deal from one locality and state to another, and patients rarely receive the entire range of services needed for satisfactory community adjustment. In addition to mental health and medical care, patients also commonly need assistance with housing, training in coping skills, supported employment, supervised activities, and social services. There are well-established programs that have been proven to be effective in providing integrated services for clients with many needs, such as the Program for Assertive Community Treatment (PACT),[34] but they typically are not available, or greatly limited, and patients in great need are commonly neglected.

Almost all care now is provided in the community, not in institutions, but most states and communities have not fulfilled the promises made with the deinstitutionalization of persons with mental illness. Vulnerable patients in the community often become involved with street drugs and other substances, in part as a way of managing their distress. Mental illness and co-occurring substance abuse is very common and complicates patients' health and the management of their care. Patients who are not properly managed increasingly fail to take their medications and get themselves into troubled situations. When their symptoms are not controlled, they are more likely to get into diffi-culty, commit legal offenses, become disturbing to the public, and become involved with the police, resulting in arrest and incarceration.

The criminalization of persons with mental illness is commonly noted, and we now have many more persons with mental illness in jails and prisons than in mental hospitals. These correctional institutions typically have poor mental health services, and persons with mental illness are commonly vic-timized by other inmates and sometimes staff. The large number of persons with mental illness in prisons is due to many factors, including poor commu-nity mental health services. But many patients are jailed for substance offenses that are by definition associated with *DSM* disorders. Moreover, neg-lected patients on the streets in impoverished and disorganized areas com-monly become involved in petty crimes and are probably less skillful than other petty criminals in avoiding detection and arrest. Efforts are being made to divert patients from the criminal justice system, to use special drug and mental health courts, to improve mental health services in jails and prisons, and to help patients reenter the community following incarceration. The prob-lems are massive, but these persons are given little priority. Much commit-ment, cooperation, and coordination between different institutions and sectors of care are needed. Achieving successful partnerships among agencies is chal-lenging and is complicated by different perspectives and values, knowledge levels, and bureaucratic interests. It is also fair to say that these patients do not fall high on the average person's hierarchy of compassion or high on political agendas. But the criminalization of the mentally ill represents per-haps the greatest scandal of our health care system, and a situation that should embarrass all thoughtful citizens.

Mental Health and Social Policy

In a refrain repeated over the decades, the President's New Freedom Commis-sion on Mental Health appointed by President George W. Bush reported that the "mental health delivery system is fragmented and in disarray."[35] The com-mission's focus properly was on care for those most seriously mentally ill, who historically have been a responsibility of government; it is these clients who depend most critically on public programs that provide medical care, housing assistance, subsistence income, supported employment, and other critical services. Persons with serious and persistent mental illness have the largest needs and are the most expensive group to provide for, but they also are a neglected population. Many receive little continuing care, are at risk of homelessness, become involved with drugs and petty crime, are jailed, and are victimized in institutions and in the community. A recent study found that 25 percent of persons with serious mental illness were victims of a violent crime in the prior year, eleven times greater than for the population as a whole.[36] Community care, as compared with custodial institutions, has brought a better life to many, perhaps most, but the public sector has persistently failed to give the care of these sickest clients sufficient priority and provide needed protections.

Part of the problem is the cost, complexity, and difficulty of building and maintaining comprehensive care arrangements that successfully integrate needed services and responsibly monitor clients. Finances are of course relevant as varying groups both in mental health and other areas of medicine jockey for public and government assistance. Priorities are confused even within the mental health sector as different subgroups compete in promoting their interests. Some intervention areas, such as prevention of mental disorder, have not been proven to be effective but have strong advocacy among influential groups and resonate with the public. Although there are many problems in providing care to seriously ill children, advocates of mental health care for children commonly focus on children and families with lesser need and on programs such as family maintenance and Drug Abuse Resistance Education (DARE) that make for better rhetoric than for effective preventive interventions. Groups that advocate in the areas of alcohol and drug abuse have their own cultures, perspectives, and service system ideas and advocate independently. The outcomes of mental health advocacy are something of a muddle, and not up to the persuasiveness of advocacy in such areas as cancer, AIDS, heart disease, and many other conditions of great public concern. One result is that when times are financially difficult in Medicaid and other government programs, services for persons with mental illness face some of the toughest restrictions.

The pharmaceutical industry is a major player on the mental health scene. As it has expanded the markets for psychiatric drugs, the industry has an increased stake in framing how mental disorders are seen and how they are treated. Through its direct-to-consumer advertising, sponsorship of psychiatric meetings, research, publications, educational activities and other events, and sponsorship of mental health advocacy groups, it seeks to expand markets and definitions of treatable mental disorders. The industry forms coalitions with advocacy groups and supports activities to extend insurance coverage for new drugs, lobbies against formularies that restrict the availability of some drugs, and seeks to persuade physicians to use its drugs "off-label," that is, for uses not specifically approved by the Food and Drug Administration. It has encouraged treatment of more people, expanding and medicalizing the mental health arena for many ordinary problems of living. Increasingly, it is apparent that the published literature on the efficacy of many new drugs is biased, since drug-company-controlled studies with less positive results may not be published and disseminated. As evidence of this has become more apparent, the editors of major medical journals have made it clear that they will not publish papers from clinical trials that have not been publicly recorded prior to initiation, so it becomes possible to monitor biased reporting of the results of drug trials.[37] The role of the pharmaceutical companies in the research process has raised troublesome questions, and this area now is receiving more attention as costs of pharmaceuticals grow much faster than other areas of medical and mental health care.

Ultimately, the role of mental health services within the health care system depends as much on values as on science, and on financial willingness to subsidize different types of treatment. While some contend that the focus should be on individuals who suffer obvious impairments from clinical disorders, others support a broader range of services to try to ameliorate disappointments and sadness, or even seek positive enhancement. It remains unclear how much positive mental enhancement is really possible with the agents now available, probably very little if any, but it is not difficult to foresee a future where new drugs will enhance the normal range of well-being, memory, and many other aspects of functioning. As with Viagra and the various other sexual enhancement drugs that followed, the public and insurers will have to decide about insurance coverage and what limits should be placed on availability.

Efforts are being made to get primary care physicians to be more attentive to their interactions with patients and to psychosocial concerns. Other professionals attached to medical practices will help with more of these activities in the future, and larger group practices will make constructive mental health management more possible, but this progress will not come quickly or easily. In recent years self-help and other support groups have taken up some of the slack, and some health plans and medical practices, as well as government, support and assist these groups in providing consumer and self-help services. Mental health concerns will continue to be handled in many ways through the general medical system, through specialty care, through self-help and consumer activities, through alternative therapies and practitioners, and through religious groups, families, and informal networks. Nevertheless, it is worrisome that almost one-third of all mental health visits in the United States are made to complementary and alternative providers in the absence of any evidence of their value.[38] One might contend that this reflects the sad state of mental health services.

As we ponder the issue of how much for whom, we must never lose sight of the smaller population of seriously impaired individuals who have traditionally been a public responsibility and who should receive first priority in our thinking and planning. This value was often violated in the last half of the twentieth century, when psychodynamic therapies dominated and interest and resources were directed commonly to those who were less sick and, in the view of many therapists, more attractive and compatible clients. As boundaries of illness expand and enhancement opportunities become viable, there is much danger that we will neglect even more those who should be our primary charge. It may seem a bit trite, but it is nevertheless true, that the quality of the system must be judged by how it treats those most vulnerable and most in need.

Chapter 5

The Activated Patient and the Doctors' Dilemma

In his book, *Overdosed America*, John Abramson, now an instructor in medicine at Harvard, describes how he explained leaving his practice after twenty years to one of his longtime patients. He relayed his frustrations with unneeded routine tests, expensive drugs that were no better or safer than older medications, and the commercial spinning of clinical decisions and scientific evidence. He explained that many of his patients, influenced by drug advertisements and the media, were increasingly visiting him with strong ideas of what they wanted and became suspicious when he tried to convert them to other interventions. He noted, "Many were reacting as if I were purposely trying to withhold the best treatment, making me choose between providing the best care and yielding to their demands in order to maintain the healing potential of our relationship."[1] Abramson defines a dilemma increasingly characteristic of relations between patients and doctors.

Traditional medical practice was highly paternalistic. Patients came with their medical complaints to doctors, who were presumably experts at diagnosis and treatment. Patients were assumed to have little knowledge and were expected to be dependent on the doctor and to be docile. In the Parsonian model of the sick role,[2] which was an influential model for many decades, patients were expected to accept their need for technically competent care, to be motivated to get well, and to cooperate in following the doctor's advice. Doctors, in turn, were to approach the patient in objective and scientifically justifiable terms and to have specifically delimited functions, defined by their expertise. They were also expected to maintain a stance of affective neutrality toward patients and to put patient welfare above their own personal interests.

Relationships were economically simple in that patients paid a fee for each encounter and doctors commonly adjusted their fees depending on patients' ability to pay.

The world of medical care is vastly different today. Patients are better educated and commonly come to doctors armed with a great deal of information and views of what they want and need. With the easy accessibility of medical information, they may already know more than the doctor about aspects of their condition, or, alternatively, have many misconceptions that need correction. Doctors are now expected to share information and options with patients and involve them in decision making. Most patients have insurance and are less concerned about cost than they were when most payments were out-of-pocket. Their physicians increasingly are also part of organized practices and influenced by payment and other incentives. Technological options for diagnosis and treatment have increased, and decisions may have important economic consequences for the doctor, patient, medical group, and health insurance plan. The economics of the encounter are no longer a simple transaction between patient and doctor but involve a variety of other parties. This chapter examines the extent to which the traditional medical care framework fits current and emerging trends, and the types of changes that are required to maintain effective doctor-patient relationships and appropriate medical professionalism.

The practice of medicine involves an array of generic functions, carried out in different ways in varying geographic contexts. Care of illness, of course, begins before people ever consult a doctor, and people deal with most symptoms and problems through informal efforts of their own, by seeking advice from relatives and friends and using over-the-counter remedies. As noted earlier, only a minority of symptoms are ever brought to medical settings. The first formal function of clinicians is to serve as doctor of first contact to assess the patients' complaints, to treat those that are less complicated and do not require more specialized assistance, to help link patients to other parts of the system and other services their conditions may require, to manage and coordinate the patients' overall health care needs, and to provide continuing management of chronic conditions after initial specialty interventions if needed. Persons performing this role are typically described as primary care physicians (PCPs) or family doctors, but in the American system this role may be performed by family doctors and general internists, pediatricians, gynecologists, or specialists in medical and surgical areas that take on primary care functions for some patients as part of their practices. Nurse practitioners, nurses, and physician assistants also often take on primary care roles. In developing nations, the primary care function is commonly performed by a range of other personnel with varying levels of training and qualifications.

The functional logic of medical care calls for a proper allocation of personnel to primary care roles, to the varying consultant specialties, and to subspecialists who provide very advanced technical services beyond those in the general specialty. In organized systems such as the English National Health Service, and in most other European countries, these functions are formally delimited by an organizational division between general practice and specialty and subspecialty care. In the American context, the distinction is informal and commonly unclear. Nevertheless, the function requires a sizable investment in primary care services, in the range of 50 percent, and smaller proportions of consulting specialist and subspecialist services. This doesn't really work out neatly in the American context because financial and other incentives discourage primary care commitments, and decreasing proportions of young doctors seek primary care careers. Thus, many people have difficulty locating doctors who take on the broad responsibilities we associate with primary care. Also, American patients resist the idea of using their general physician as a gateway to more specialized care and often seek such care directly. Once having established a relationship with a specialist, the patient may choose to return to that specialist for the continuing management of a long-term condition. When managed care organizations sought to require patients to receive a referral from their primary care physician prior to specialty care, many patients were unhappy, which contributed to the managed care backlash. And, as noted, many specialists fill in their schedules by providing basic primary care services to some of their patients.

The specialty organization of American medicine can be seen as a central, implicit policy that defines how we carry out our medical affairs.[3] The specialties and their societies are private organizations, but they play a major role in self-regulation of the profession, specialty certification, graduate medical education, and matters such as testing for competence, promoting quality improvement, reimbursement, and recruitment needs. As part of an interlocking set of organizations involved in educational and practice issues, the specialty societies constitute a major private part of the private/public system of professional regulation. There are twenty-four medical specialty boards under the dominant American Board of Medical Specialties (ABMS), and some competitive organizations that also provide certifications. The ABMS certifies thirty-seven primary specialties, and these specialty organizations provide certification for a growing number of subspecialties now numbering ninety-two. Almost all doctors (including family physicians) are certified as specialists of some sort, and these boards now certify almost 90 percent of all practicing physicians.[4] Subspecialties are being added at a rapid rate, with sixty-four new additions since 1980. The most recent specialty group, added in 1991, was the American Board of Medical Genetics, and other groups aspire to reach board status. There is no inherent system logic in this organizational proliferation other than to break medical tasks into smaller and smaller units representing the growing knowledge and technological base. But it is also a source of fragmentation and failures in coordination. Certification serves as a basis for attracting patients and demanding higher fees.

Efforts have been made over decades to increase the supply of primary care physicians, but the condition of primary care continues to erode.[5] Perhaps most influential are financial incentives that reward specialists far more than PCPs. Some efforts have been made to close the gap between payment for procedures and tests, which reward specialists handsomely, and payment for thoughtful listening, communication, instruction, and behavioral services, characteristic of primary care, which are challenging but pay relatively little. Still, there is little willingness to pay for the real time that doctors must spend to counsel patients and involve them meaningfully in their own care. In addition, specialists have greater prestige and typically have more control over their time than PCPs, who are expected to maintain a continuing and more personal relationship with their patients. Also, given the value placed on technological advance in American society, and the dominant value system in medicine, those who provide what are viewed as more mundane services of everyday medical care are seen as less accomplished and are in some cases less valued by their colleagues. Much of what primary care doctors do is seen among medical peers as routine and intellectually uninteresting.

Primary care is challenging and exciting if doctors work seriously with patients to address the social and behavioral factors that affect illness and adherence to an appropriate regimen and to enhance self-care and health maintenance, but these tasks are honored more in rhetoric than in reality. It doesn't take acute perception to understand that the more tangible rewards follow those who pursue the subspecialist route. Median income for primary care doctors in the year 2003 was $157,000, compared with just under $300,000 for all specialists. Specialists varied from $163,000 for psychiatrists and $191,000 for neurologists, low-paid specialists, to $410,000 for invasive cardiologists.[6] Despite lower incomes, many doctors are drawn to primary care because of their interest in people and their aspirations to practice a more holistic approach to medicine than specialty care typically allows.

Many studies over the years have shown that well-organized primary care is intrinsic to an effective system of health care.[7] The management of most illnesses, and almost all preventive care needs, can be handled capably and routinely within a primary care relationship that offers access to care, health monitoring, coordination with other needed services, and instructional and support services. Primary care provides the opportunity to use resources thoughtfully with limited duplication, fragmentation, and breakdowns in communication, and the effective use of clinical teams to achieve defined preventive and disease management objectives. Studies in the United States and around the world have repeatedly found that medical care organized around strong primary care systems is associated with favorable illness and mortality outcomes.[8] In particular instances specialist care may be more expert and evidence based than care provided at the primary care level, but most care can be provided capably and cost-effectively as part of the routine longitudinal management of the patient. Indeed, effective primary care brings to bear knowledge of the patients's entire medical situation and often protects against unnecessary and even harmful interventions when the focus is the disease and not the patient.

Even in limited medical circumstances when few resources are available, as is characteristic of many poor countries and impoverished areas in the United States, organizing a frontline system of care that is accessible, deals with basic preventive care such as immunizations and maternal and child care, treats common health problems, and provides health guidance, contributes immensely to population health outcomes. Greater resources and more developed primary care offer further opportunities through sophisticated diagnostic and treatment facilities and teams to address not only acute care issues but also issues of health maintenance, effective functioning, rehabilitation, and behavioral health. Our problem is not that we lack understanding of how to do these things but rather that competing interests and incentives make implementation difficult and encourage physicians and others to direct their interest and attention to more lucrative opportunities.

Enter the Activated Patient

"Consumerism" has become a significant buzzword in health care, although people have different concepts of what this means. Those seeking to establish a more viable medical marketplace see increased consumer involvement as a means to increase competition among health care plans in providing the price, service, and quality of care mix that consumers most prefer. They believe that providing more information to consumers about health plan performance will allow consumers to signal through their choices how they want their health care structured and to influence plans competing for patients. This remains an important aspiration, but there is little evidence that patients have such clout. Consumers seem most attuned to cost issues, and health plans do better economically by avoiding the sickest and most expensive patients than by expanding services and focusing on excellence. In fact, being an outlier on quality often attracts sicker patients, the cost of whose care and treatment, in health plans with fixed, prospective premiums and payments, often puts providers and plans at a financial disadvantage.

Many consumer groups organized around diseases seek to inform members and involve them in pressuring government, health plans, and provider groups to finance and organize services particular to their needs. Consumer groups have succeeded in substantially revising obstetrical care and child delivery, AIDS research and treatment, breast cancer treatment, and some services for persons with serious mental illness. Each major disease group now has its consumer and professional constituencies, which compete for attention, financial support, and increased priority. Consumerism is also active in the proliferation of self-help and illness support groups whose participants share information and advise each other about treatments, sympathetic professionals and provider groups, and means of coping with their condition. Then there are the millions of people, affiliated with no formal group, who troll the Internet for health information and who participate in health and disease chat groups.

Consumerism takes place in an entrepreneurial context. Pharmaceutical companies, health plans, technology companies and hospitals among others seek to influence how consumers view disease and medical treatments. In the year 2001, for example, the pharmaceutical industry reported that it spent $19.1 billion dollars on marketing, most of it targeting physicians directly, but also including $2.7 billion for direct-to-consumer (DTC) advertising.[9] Marcia Angell, former editor of the *New England Journal of Medicine*, has analyzed these data and argues that a more accurate estimate is $54 billion constituting 30 percent of members of the Pharmaceutical Research and Manufacturers of America's (PhRMA) $179 billion in revenues in 2001.[10] Expenditures on DTC almost tripled between 1997 and 2001, with television ads accounting for almost two-thirds of such advertising.[11] This vast DTC expenditure is relatively small compared with the massive funds spent on direct promotion to physicians by sales representatives, and through a variety of techniques from providing free drug samples and knickknacks to promoting drugs through sponsorship of continuing education. The *Industry Profile* reports that companies employ far more people for marketing (86,226) than for research and development (51,589).[12]

The efforts to influence consumers and their physician agents is very big business. Pharmaceutical companies fund consumer groups and team up with them in efforts to lobby state Medicaid programs and others to add new expensive drugs that have not been shown to be superior to less expensive generic drugs to drug formularies. In its quest to gain brand allegiance and increased sales, the pharmaceutical industry is a major presence at meetings of almost every medical professional organization as a significant sponsor of their activities, happily providing gifts small and large, and lucrative consultancies for major figures.[13] Thus it seeks to influence not only the drugs patients ask for but, even more, the inclinations of physicians to provide those drugs. Much is at stake in the choices physicians make under ordinary prescribing circumstances, which explains why so much marketing is directed at physicians. Drug expenditures are larger than necessary as physicians prescribe expensive new drugs that are often no better, and sometimes less effective and more dangerous, than inexpensive generic alternatives. There is some case to be made that DTC advertising may alert people to treatments from which they could benefit and make it less stigmatizing to seek assistance, but the overall influence of pharmaceutical industry advertising has added vast expense with little demonstrated advantage. As editors of major medical journals have learned, it is increasingly difficult to identify persons who have appropriate expertise to review pharmaceuticals who do not have significant potential conflicts of interest because of consultancies with the industry.

Although the pharmaceutical industry is the most obvious player, similar efforts are made to promote new untested treatments, appliances and devices, disease management programs, health promotion programs, and even practice guidelines. The new activated consumer is caught in an advertising blitz from many sides, making it extremely difficult to ascertain what is true and what is hype. The agencies consumers presumably rely on, perhaps most importantly the Food and Drug Administration (FDA), lack the authority and resources to match the hucksterism of the American medical scene. Although consumers generally have little trust in government, the FDA had developed a reputation of trustworthiness associated with its success in the 1960s in keeping thalidomide off the market; the drug resulted in many deformed children in other countries. In efforts to increase the pace of drug approvals, which critics argued was delaying the introduction of important drugs, the FDA accelerated its pace of drug reviews in 1992, financed substantially by contributions from the pharmaceutical companies; some believe this focus on approving drugs more quickly and its commercial support and related influence have led to taking more risks than desirable. That is, of course, debatable, but American consumers generally do not understand that the FDA only assesses whether new drugs are safe and efficacious, not whether they are superior or even comparable to drugs already on the market. Many "me-too" drugs capture high market share through advertising and promotion to physicians rather than superior performance.[14] Consumers also do not understand the limits on the FDA in post-marketing monitoring of approved drugs whose long-term negative effects are often not clear until many people have used the drug and been harmed. The findings on the cardiovascular effects of Cox-2 inhibitors that resulted in the withdrawal from the market of Vioxx and Bextra, two blockbuster drugs (see the introduction of this book), have made the need for improved post-marketing surveillance more apparent. The negative publicity and subsequent congressional pressure that resulted from the problems with the Cox-2 inhibitors have resulted in a slowing of new drug approvals by the FDA.

When in doubt, even the most sophisticated patients look to their physicians for guidance, because they have more trust in their doctors than in many of the other sources of information available to them. Although ideally physicians should be in a position to make meaningful judgments, this too often is an unrealistic expectation. Physicians have busy lives and limited time to critically review the enormous pharmaceutical literature. They depend more than is desirable on drug detail representatives, advertising, and hype. They typically do not know how drugs within major classes compare in terms of relative costs, or the insurance coverage of their patients. Thus, they fall victim to the same promotional influences that consumers do.

Some help is underway through an effort by Consumers Union, working with physician consultants, to provide patients with information about the relative costs and benefits of frequently used drugs in a user-friendly fashion, with comparative cost data and recommendations of best buys. Seven reports on such commonly used medications as antidepressants, statins, and blood pressure drugs have been issued and are available free on the web at www.CRBestBuyDrugs.org. Four more reports are in the process of being compiled as this is being written, and more are planned. The cost information in these reports is particularly valuable for individuals who must pay for their own drugs, perhaps less so for those who are part of large drug plans that may receive discounts on many brand name medications. A report in *JAMA* on this development notes that physicians working with the program believe that the reports could also be valuable clinical tools for physicians, by providing reliable information on drug options and comparative costs.[15]

Computerized support systems can remedy some informational deficiencies by providing real-time feedback to doctors on issues of drug efficacy, side effects, cost, and drug interactions. But these systems are expensive, and most physician groups are reluctant to spend the money for them. Drug formularies can help as well, but pharmaceutical companies fight such formularies and have many strategies, such as mobilizing consumers and creating special pricing arrangements, for getting their drugs included.

Despite the barriers, many physicians take a scientific perspective in their prescribing and make efforts to educate their patients about the value and cost-effectiveness of alternative treatments and drugs. When patients come in asking for an advertised drug, the doctor uses the occasion to inform them, perhaps directing them to a better treatment regimen or a more appropriate medication and using the occasion as a learning opportunity. One recent physician survey found that doctors believed that DTC advertising led patients to seek unnecessary treatments, but physicians sometimes used these occasions to suggest other treatments or lifestyle changes.[16] Physician respondents reported that they prescribed the requested drug about two-fifths of the time. In about half the cases, they believed the requested drug would have no overall health effect, but they were influenced by a desire to please the patient.

The Doctors' Dilemma

Physicians seeking to practice a high level of professionalism in these matters face two significant barriers. They typically have limited time for each patient. Making patients partners in care and spending time educating them is a worthy endeavor that physicians commonly support, but they fear the difficulties of interrupting their practice pace and getting off schedule. Reeducating the patient can be a time-consuming process with a determined patient, and it is often much easier to agree to a patient's request, if it would do no apparent harm, than to get into extended controversies.[17] Also, doctors realize that some patients are determined to get what they want and will go to another doctor if their request is refused. Most doctors these days are not ready to antagonize and lose patients, particularly those that have good insurance and aren't particularly troublesome.

Although the time expended in the typical patient visit has increased in the past couple of decades and now averages fifteen to twenty minutes,[18] the demands on doctors have increased even more, leaving them with a feeling that there isn't sufficient time for doing all that should be done.[19] Lack of time is one of the most persistent complaints in physician surveys, and this has been the case for decades. Physicians often have more control over their time than their survey responses suggest, so the perception of lack of time must be interpreted in the context of income. Physicians commonly view time expenditures in relation to an expected target income. Physicians could spend more time with their patients if they were willing to forego the additional income they would get from seeing more patients during the time period allotted. Doctors are no longer able to charge whatever they like for a patient visit, so under typical insurance, time becomes money. A small number of doctors have concierge practices that require a monthly or yearly retainer in addition to their fees, and they promise patients more time and other amenities. This may work for physicians who dislike the typical pace of practice and wish to practice in a fashion they view as more optimal, but few physicians can realistically expect to develop a sufficient clientele of such paying patients. Such preferential service practices also are undesirable from a social point of view because they enlarge rather than close inequalities. Many believe that while such preferences might be appropriate for other areas of living, we should strive for greater equality in medical care.

Given a fixed expenditure of time, physicians face escalating and competing expectations. There are increasingly more treatments to choose from, requiring not only careful thought but time to explain options to patients. Physicians are also expected to give attention to many facets of prevention, including immunization, smoking cessation, diet, exercise, and sexual behavior. A recent study found that if physicians followed all the recommended preventive care guidelines of the U.S. Preventive Services Task Force, they would have little time for all else.[20] It is no surprise that studies repeatedly find that many of the more complex preventive activities are typically not done, and even the simple ones are often neglected.[21] Also, the boundaries of medical work continue to expand, encompassing many of the common problems of living. As I noted earlier, promoters of drugs, new technologies, and other interventions have strong motivation to define new diseases and body enhancements that can provide a market for their wares. Some of these have value and some don't, but there is much to explain to patients who believe a product is something they might benefit from. And, of course, there are increasing numbers of patients seeking services, armed with information from DTC advertising, the Internet, and other media sources.

Payers as well as patients have expectations. Physicians are increasingly required to participate in quality-assurance activities, provide information required by health plans, and cooperate in other ways in efforts to increase quality and make care more cost-effective. Complex insurance payment arrangements and the many complexities associated with multiple health plans require much attention to administrative matters. Although most physicians have office staff that do most of this type of work for them, there is inevitably some burden. Office staff also require monitoring and supervision. One of the major lapses in medical groups is the poor training and supervision of employees who deal with patients. Large medical groups may have appropriate office management staff, but smaller practices often do not. Physicians themselves have little incentive to become involved in practice management: it is not financially advantageous, typically not much fun, and often leads to disputes with one's colleagues and others.[22] Hospitals also make new demands in responding to quality-assurance needs, efforts to reduce medical error, and cost problems. Doctors are expected to be more accountable than they have been in the past.

Finally, while managed care strategies are not as intrusive and difficult for doctors as they once were, some time inevitably must be spent in justifying treatments and particular patient needs. These expectations are made more burdensome by the fact that physicians must deal with many different health plans, each having its own requirements, procedures, and information needs. It is no surprise that some physicians report that they feel as if life is a treadmill, and that quality and performance studies find that much is left undone.

Although care partnerships are touted as the desirable practice arrangement and there is much rhetoric about partnerships, the concept itself is not well defined, and the reality is hard to find except perhaps in some academic settings where time pressures are less evident, or in specialized settings such as cancer treatment centers. Most thoughtful observers interested in the concept believe that it requires patient visits of approximately half an hour, a time allocation that, given medical and economic realities, is unlikely in general primary care practices. Needless to say, there are what economists call opportunity costs. While there is much evidence that effective and continuing primary care partnership relationships contribute to higher quality of care and greater patient adherence to medical advice,[23] it is not so clear that increasing doctor-patient visit time by 50 to 100 percent is the best way to use physician time, or that it constitutes a cost-effective approach. Advocates for such partnerships rarely examine the cost implications relative to alternative ways of achieving similar objectives. In any case, widespread partnerships are unlikely except perhaps in some specialty care niches and in adaptations like concierge practice.

The Role of Professionalism and Medical Organization

It is easy to understand how practice pressures push doctors toward the easier route of accommodating to patient requests rather than making the more demanding educational effort, but this is the antithesis of the professionalism that medicine aspires to promote. The professional responsibility is to serve as an expert and guide, not all-knowing and dogmatic, but open to exploration and meaningful negotiation. If the physician is simply to give patients what they want, regardless of judgments of effectiveness and value, it can hardly be said that the physician is functioning in a professional manner. Values may vary a great deal from one person and group to another. Professionalism is not an imposition of one's values on others. What is required is understanding patients' requests in light of their own values and life goals, and providing them with the best possible guidance within their own frames of reference. Studies of patient decision making find that patients given adequate explanations of their options commonly make decisions that are different from those their physician might choose.[24] The role of the physician is to ensure that the patient understands the costs and benefits of alternative decisions, not to decide for the patient unless the patient wishes the physician to do so.

Given the realities of doctors' income aspirations, the many demands on their time, and the increased focus on rising costs and the need for cost constraints, much of the discussion about partnerships and holistic care seems unrealistic. It appears unlikely that the professional and educational goals that advocates aspire to can be achieved within the existing financial and practice structures. Medicine requires a different way of doing its business.

Significant advances have taken place in some large, well-organized medical care programs, such as the Kaiser Permanente Medical Groups[25] and the Veterans Affairs[26] system, in promoting a new kind of professionalism built around evidence-based collegial processes and quality-assurance programs supported by advanced information technology, well-developed disease management programs, and teams of supporting professionals. Some maintain that we have to rediscover the logic of the traditional prepaid organized health practice that provides a template for implementing many of the new approaches to professional practice that are responsive to emerging challenges.[27] The fact is, however, that most medical practices remain small and loosely organized, and there is little push from health plans, professionals, or patients to move toward these more organized systems of care.[28] Implementation of practice improvement, at least in the foreseeable future, has to be achieved through virtual networks, collaborations, alliances, and other less formal organizational strategies.

For typical physicians in small practices throughout the country, faced with all the pressures already described, the efforts and commitments required seem excessive. Even something as obvious as computerizing one's practice and putting in place computerized systems for improved patient care seems formidable. First there are the start-up costs and learning costs, which require more than the usual investment of money and time. Small practices are unlikely to have individuals on hand to troubleshoot and to address new issues as they develop. And maintaining the systems take effort, intelligence, and input time. There are of course many vendors offering a range of systems and services, but choosing among them and then having systems that are compatible with affiliated institutions can be difficult. Physicians in small practices lacking information technology (IT) expertise look at the challenges and conclude it is not worth the trouble and financial cost, and they see no one willing to pay for the time invested in using and maintaining these systems intelligently. Although the value of IT for improving care and assisting effective clinical decision making has been well documented, cost savings have yet to be convincingly demonstrated.[29]

Given the reality that we are unlikely to have either more large, organized groups, which many physicians and patients dislike, or the extensive consolidation of payers and plans that would make implementation of innovation more likely, we jump from one inadequate initiative to another. With so many different actors trying to call the shots, physicians often find that the most comfortable adaptation is to persist in what has seemed to work. The problem isn't so much that we are ignorant of the changes needed but more that the politics of making them are so formidable.

Consider some of the issues already discussed. Consistent implementation is impossible when each health plan has its own preferences and guidelines and no one can speak for the profession. In some locations, plans come together to agree on a common format, but this is more the exception than the norm. Pharmaceutical companies spend massive amounts to influence (they say educate) physicians about drugs and consumers about treatments. It would be sensible to tax all pharmaceuticals and have this informational function performed by an agency that reviews the evidence objectively and disseminates accurate information to doctors and patients. Such public "detailing" has been advocated for decades and has been proven to work successfully,[30] but it is hard to imagine the politics that could make it a reality in the United States. Other health systems, like the English National Health Service, have agencies such as the National Institute for Health and Clinical Excellence (NICE)[31] whose role is to provide advice to the NHS and encourage doctors to use medications in a more evidence-based way, and the NHS uses its large buying power to bargain over price of pharmaceuticals. In contrast, the recent Medicare bill that extended pharmaceutical coverage explicitly forbade the government from using its purchasing power to keep drug prices down.

There is no quick fix in the American context for the practice and quality issues that are of concern. However, for the most part physicians are a highly select and well-trained group who aspire to take good care of their patients. They seek to do well while doing good, but they face increasing demands and extraordinary pressures, and function in an environment of information overload, with many seeking to influence them. The older professional orientation built around clinical responsibility and individual autonomy no longer fits the changing environment of accelerating knowledge and technology, financial and organizational changes, and new consumer activism. Nor does it fit the corporate influences from health plans and pharmaceutical companies and the constraints imposed by government regulation. There are signs of a budding new professionalism, better matched to contemporary conditions, but it remains underdeveloped and difficult to implement across the board.

Many influences can contribute to the maturation of a new professionalism, but there are difficult political battles to be fought to get there. Central to promoting professionalism is assuring that doctors get the most advanced and most reliable information that assists decision making, unbiased by marketing and special interest. Various organizations around the world are now attempting to build helpful databases such as the nonprofit Cochrane Collaboration, which enlists thousands of physicians and health scientists to bring together what we have learned about various treatments from controlled trials.[32] Legal changes that would require the FDA to assess how new pharmaceutical entities perform relative to existing drugs, rather than just their safety and superiority relative to placebos, would constitute a major advance.[33] Enacting and financing a system of public pharmaceutical detailing that gives physicians objective guidance on safety and effectiveness of medications and provides guidance to the public as well would be a countervailing influence to pharmaceutical promotion.

It takes some effort and discernment to make sense of the enormous output of health research in the United States and around the world. The budget of the National Institutes of Health, the main U.S. biomedical research agency, was almost $29 billion in 2005, but most of it was for basic research. The pharmaceutical industry spends a comparable amount but funds most clinical trials to satisfy FDA requirements and to bring drugs to market. Increasingly, the industry depends on private contract research organizations rather than academic researchers to carry out these studies, but in either case it exercises a great deal of influence over these trials. Unfavorable results may be buried rather than published, or reported in such a way as to mislead reviewers and editors. Some clinical trials are used primarily for marketing rather than to inform standards of care. In 2001, editors of more than a dozen prestigious journals around the world, including the *New England Journal of Medicine*, *JAMA*, and *The Lancet*, attempted to address these abuses and issued strengthened requirements for research publications. They noted in their original editorial that "the use of clinical trials primarily for marketing, in our view, makes a mockery of clinical investigation and is a misuse of a powerful tool."[34] They also strongly criticized many of the controls that pharmaceutical sponsors exercised over the design of trials and publication. Marcia Angell, a former editor of the *New England Journal of Medicine*, notes that she increasingly saw "companies begin to exercise a level of control over the way research is done . . . and the aim was clearly to load the dice to make sure their drugs looked good."[35] We lack sufficient countervailing influence to help the public, and even practicing doctors, make sense of clinical trial results in the onslaught of pharmaceutical promotion.

While United States medicine is not organized in a way that allows the type of full court press taking place in the United Kingdom to improve the capacities of primary care, we can do much more than at present. We can facilitate the computerization of medical practices and the development of compatible systems so communication across practices is more possible, provide technical assistance to develop appropriate electronic medical records and deal with privacy issues, and put in place aids to improve practice and avoid errors. It is already apparent that individual interests such as pharmaceutical companies and health plans are ready to offer their assistance in exchange for access to databases and physician allegiance, contributing still another layer to the conflict of interest that plagues American health care. Both government and medical professional organizations have to take a proactive role in helping practices build systems independent of such special interests. In July 2005, it was reported that Medicare would provide electronic health record software free to help physicians computerize their medical practices, an important step. The software is a version of Vista, a well-developed system used by Veterans Affairs health facilities and associated with the improvements in care made in recent years at those facilities. Doctors may still require considerable technical help in implementing and learning to use this system, and those in private practice may prefer systems better aligned with billing needs. Professional medical organizations also have to play a more positive role and separate themselves from the kinds of industry sponsorship that compromise their independence and medical professionalism.[36]

None of this is going to be easy, and it is impossible to divorce medical practice from the historical, cultural, and economic context within which it functions. American medicine is a big business, and marketing interests and entrepreneurial motivations are evident at every turn. We can rail against corporate influence, commercialization, and profit orientations, but it is naive to expect these influences to be superceded. Professionals and their organizations, with the help of nonprofit organizations and government, can do a great deal to constrain these influences, reduce conflicts of interest, and bring a higher level of professionalism and ethical behavior to the mix. Thus, we have some chance to garner the ingenuity and innovativeness of an incentivized pluralistic marketplace while tempering some of its more extreme and undesirable side effects. A reactivated medical professionalism can be a powerful buffer between marketing excesses and the welfare of patients. Promoting such professionalism, however challenging, is a worthy endeavor.

Chapter 6

The Neglect of Long-Term Care

Many of us who have experienced the deterioration and death of parents or loved ones when the care process breaks down, as it often does at the end of life, share some sense of helplessness and frustration. Being an experienced medical professional doesn't necessarily help, because even expertise cannot counterbalance faulty systems that work against you. In a moving essay, Jerald Winakur, a geriatrician with thirty years experience and the medical director of a hospital skilled-nursing unit, describes his sense of loss and futility as his elderly father became increasingly disabled and demented. As Winakur notes, all of the complications of disability and confusion are compounded by the "sad and frustrating fact that our government appears to have no policy vision for long-term elder care."[1] He describes a stream of seemingly intractable problems, including the lack of long-term custodial care coverage except for the destitute, the dangers of hospital care for the elderly with likelihood of significant errors, and the simple fact that doctors faced with many "sexy" career choices have little motivation to care for elderly people on an inevitably downward course. There are thirty-five million people age sixty-five and over and almost five million age eighty-five or older in the United States, but only nineteen hundred doctors are credentialed in long-term care.

A major challenge to our health care system is to adapt more appropriately to the challenge of chronic disease and to better manage patients so as to minimize disabilities and maximize effective function. As the population continues to age, the already large numbers of persons with chronic disease and with multiple conditions will continue to mount. There is heartening evidence that as each successive population cohort ages, disabilities are delayed until later in life, but skeptics note that advances have been primarily in areas called instrumental activities of daily living, such as managing one's finances or using the telephone, which may have been made easier by new technologies such as phones with large numbers and buttons, enhanced sound capacities, voice-activated calling, and redial features. This is in contrast, for example, to toileting or bathing, where new technologies are more modest. Whatever future studies find about age and disability, the growing numbers of older people with chronic disease and disabilities will provide abundant work that stretches the resources of the health care system.

Chronic-care management becomes increasingly problematic as patients become frailer and acquire multiple illnesses and disabilities that seriously impede function and lead to impairments in performance in the activities of daily living. It is at this point that persons require long-term-care services. Long-term-care services in the United States are expensive, difficult to organize and coordinate, insufficiently comprehensive, and do not do a good enough job of meeting the needs of elders, families, and other informal caregivers. To make a bad situation worse, the care is of uneven quality across settings, whether in nursing homes, assisted care facilities, foster care homes, patients' own homes, or elsewhere in the community. Doctors and nurses try hard despite poorly organized care arrangements to take good care of persons with chronic diseases and disabilities, but they are thwarted by the difficulty of implementing well-designed disease-management approaches and by limited opportunities for effective use of multidisciplinary approaches and teams.

Long-term care in the United States is the stepchild of our health care system, and it exhibits, even in more extreme ways, many of the difficulties and deficiencies that characterize health care more generally. Clients in long-term care typically have multiple diseases and disabilities and difficulty in caring fully for themselves because of limitations in function. They require not only good medical care but also rehabilitation services, and much attention to social circumstances and needed social supports.

Promoting effective health and functioning in this population requires attention to an array of needs, from attentive medical care and careful medication management to such other issues as nutrition and appropriate diet, exercise, physical and occupational therapy, social activities, and psychological support. Among older cohorts, cognitive decline is more apparent, and increasing numbers suffer from confusion and dementias, making these persons more difficult to manage and requiring caretakers with special skills and empathy.[2] It is not uncommon for these patients to be stigmatized and neglected, especially when they lack support and attention from loved ones. It is

sad, but nevertheless true, that many if not most of the persons with the greatest need do not get the expert attention and high-quality management they
require.

To be sure, innumerable papers, reports, proposals, and exposés have illu-
minated the long-term care crisis.[3] But few policy makers are prepared to
address this problem, not because of disinterest or lack of concern, but because
of worries about potential cost. Long-term care is largely an informal system in
which people struggle along with the assistance of family and friends, predominantly daughters and other women. Perhaps as much as 80 percent of care
is provided through informal networks. Long-term care typically is not seen as
a core part of medical care, and most health insurance plans do not cover most
vital long-term-care services except for short periods as part of care for an acute
medical episode.

A private long-term-care insurance sector has been developing over the
past couple of decades, but it faces many difficulties and uncertainties, and
modest enrollment. Purchasers have some difficulty understanding exactly
what would be covered and how adequate it will be in the future, given
expected rising prices. The insurance costs seem relatively expensive when
purchased for services that people might or might not need in the seemingly
distant future. Moreover, middle-aged persons with modest incomes and no
large assets to protect must weigh these future needs among many current ones
that may seem more pressing. Purchasers also face many other uncertainties.
Will the insurers still be in business when they need care? What happens to
their investment if they are unable to afford their premiums for a year or two?
How can they be assured that the determination of their medical eligibility,
when the time comes, will be fair? Will their options or choices be limited in
unforeseen ways? Insurers also have difficulty predicting future long-term-care
costs and restrict coverage in various ways; they may charge premiums that
seem excessive to protect themselves against future losses. Also, it is not clear
that long-term-care insurance is a good choice for people of modest means,
since they are likely to become eligible for Medicaid or other public support
should they develop major long-term-care needs. Thus, most people who
require such assistance fall back on their own resources and those of their
loved ones, and mostly on informal sources of assistance.

Efforts by state governments and by interested foundations such as The
Robert Wood Johnson Foundation (RWJF) have been made to expand the
long-term-care insurance market but with limited success.[4] The RWJF, for
example, set up a partnership for long-term care involving four states as far
back as 1988. This effort sought to induce people to purchase private long-

term care insurance by offering as an incentive less stringent eligibility criteria for Medicaid once the private benefits had been exhausted. This essentially offered enrollees asset protection should they need to go onto Medicaid (Medicaid enrollees under usual circumstances can keep only the most modest assets). This was a clever conceptual idea, but, despite much effort, relatively few private policies were purchased.

When individuals have exhausted their personal resources, Medicaid is their safety net. Medicaid is not only the largest health care program in the United States but also America's de facto long-term-care program, and it pays for about half of all nursing home care. About 40 percent of nursing home residents had Medicaid as the expected source of payment when admitted, but many who enter nursing homes with their own resources exhaust them quickly and also gain eligibility. Thus, Medicaid is the expected source of payment of three-fifths of nursing home residents.[5] Medicaid, as a federal-state partnership, gives states considerable discretion to extend services beyond required elements. Thus, eligibility and benefits covered may vary a great deal depending on where one lives. Some states invest half or more of Medicaid expenditures in long-term care, while others invest very little. In 2000, New York and Connecticut invested an average of $14,000 per year for each eligible elderly person, while South Carolina, Mississippi, and Oklahoma spent less than $5,000. Medicaid long-term care remains very much institutionally based, with two-thirds of expenditures as late as 2003 still going to institutions despite the focus on delivering more long-term care in the home and community. Most elderly persons fear nursing homes and do anything possible to avoid them, and this reluctance has served naturally to control demand and ration services.

Nevertheless, there has been progress as efforts have been made by various states to bring more long-term-care services into the client's home and other community-based residences such as group homes and assisted-living facilities. This is reflected by the reduction of Medicaid long-term expenditures for institutional care from 87 percent to 70 percent between 1990 and 2002.[6] Some states, notably Oregon, have been innovative in providing most long-term care in community-based settings that are less restrictive than nursing homes and more consistent with client preference; options include home care, foster home residence, and other forms of assisted living.[7] A significant Supreme Court decision in a mental health case (*Olmstead v. L.C.*, 1999) in a lawsuit brought under the Americans with Disabilities Act, is helping push toward providing community-based alternatives under Medicaid by supporting clients' rights to receive long-term care in less restrictive environments. Many states have commissions and other work groups seeking to develop compliance plans. The difficult fiscal problems faced by states in recent years has been slowing the process.[8] As with many such legal decisions, it will take a decade or more for the implications to play out, but *Olmstead* provides the impetus for states to plan differently about how Medicaid will be administered in the future.

It has always been clear that most clients have preferred to receive long-term-care assistance in home and in more personalized community settings, but policy makers resisted because they feared much increased demand. They understood that most community long-term-care services were being provided informally and without economic cost to the public, and they worried that should more eligible people use public services, costs would be transferred to taxpayers. Concerned with the growth of their Medicaid budgets, states monitor eligibility for services closely and provide services sparingly. Studies as part of demonstration projects that examined the feared cost shift found that, contrary to expectation, public community-based services complemented informal care rather than replaced it.[9] Many clients in public programs do not receive anywhere near what they really need, and the public/private mix produces a more appropriate and responsive care pattern. Over the years, we have also learned much about how caregiving to persons with high levels of need, such as those with Alzheimer's disease and other significant disabilities, have high personal costs for the caregivers, who suffer much stress, restricted lives, and related health problems. Transfer of some long-term-care burdens to the public sector sometimes is the sensible and appropriate course of action.

There has been much discussion of home- and community-based alternatives under Medicaid, but, as already noted, the program remains substantially institutionally based. Part of the problem is the legal framework of Medicaid, which requires states to provide institutional services but leaves decisions about home and community services to states' discretion. Fearing escalation of their already mounting Medicaid costs, states tend to fund nursing home alternatives through federal waivers that allow them to limit where and to whom these services will be available. Many states are reported to have waiting lists for home- and community-based services, which is simply another way of rationing services and controlling expenditures. In the private sector there has been large growth of life-care communities, offering various levels of assisted care as need develops, but such communities are mainly organized for middle-class persons with sufficient assets to pay significant entrance fees and monthly maintenance. Nevertheless, there has been significant growth in the emerging assisted-living industry. There is no agreed-upon definition of assisted living, or national data on clients, but informed observers believe that approximately one million clients now receive some level of assisted living, most financing their care with their own resources. In contrast, most persons of limited means must depend more on public support and public programs, which typically do not pay for residence in assisted-living facilities. There are no definitive studies, but anecdotal information and the impressions of many experts suggest that assisted-care settings range widely in quality and intensity of assistance and are often less than adequate.

Over the past twenty years a number of efforts have been made to develop long-term-care programs that integrate acute medical care and long-term-care services under capitation-type arrangements.[10] These programs have been based on the belief that an integrated approach that provides essential long-term-care services when they are needed will result in less use of acute medical care and fewer unneeded expensive medical interventions with the elderly. On-Lok, an important capitated model, dates back to the 1970s. On-Lok organized integrated services (including housing, nutrition, day care, and other services) for a poor, frail, elderly Chinese population in San Francisco and seemed to have considerable success. This inspired the Centers for Medicare and Medicaid Services (CMS), then known as the Health Care Financing Administration (HCFA), to develop PACE (Program of All Inclusive Care for the Elderly) as a demonstration under authorization of the Omnibus Budget Reconciliation Act of 1986. Like On-Lok, PACE targeted persons eligible for nursing home care who wished to remain in the community. Following an interdisciplinary approach, it sought to integrate social and medical services through organizations that function like staff HMOs. The capitation is basically constructed by integrating Medicare and Medicaid funding. After its initial success as a demonstration project, PACE was made permanent as a Medicare program under the Balanced Budget Act (BBA) of 1997.[11]

Advocates still remain enthusiastic about this model, and the effort continues, but PACE remains a very small program. The BBA authorized 180 non-profit and 10 for-profit PACE programs, but by the end of 2002 there were only 39 programs in place serving about 10,000 clients. PACE requires clients to participate in adult day care and use care providers associated with the program, features not particularly attractive to many elderly people who are reluctant to change doctors, and enrollment has been difficult. There are many other barriers to implementing these programs.[12] Few who actually enroll leave the program, but PACE will have to become a much larger program to have significant impact.

A related effort called the Social Health Maintenance Organization (SHMO) was developed to expand HMOs by adding various long-term-care services such as personal care, homemaking, case management, and meals. Initially, there were four demonstration sites. SHMOs were to be put to a competitive market test in which both unimpaired and impaired elderly had to pay increased premiums for a program that would cover some long-term-care needs. The idea was that through coordinated case management, disability criteria would be applied to assess need and services would be authorized as required. The demonstration encountered serious marketing and implementation problems that added to cost. Although the demonstration found that SHMOs could control use of expanded services and costs, acute medical care costs were higher than expected.[13] Many policy makers lost interest, and the concept never gained momentum. Informally, among health policy experts, some believe that the name, Social Health Maintenance Organization, itself, dissonant with emerging dominant ideologies, helped sink the concept.

As with much in public policy intervention, simplicity helps, and complicated, integrated organized interventions are difficult to sustain and implement widely across plans and providers. Thus, simpler ideas like long-term care in foster homes or residential care facilities, and subsidizing relatives for providing some long-term care are a lot easier to implement than complex new organizational approaches that seek to integrate services across many areas of care. Having been involved in several such efforts in the treatment of mental illness, I know how difficult it is to turn theory into reality, particularly when efforts require bringing together varying organizational bureaucracies with different priorities, cultures, and systems of rewards for participants.[14] There is a tendency for each new governmental administration to announce presumably new and exciting initiatives that will change things, but most never amount to much unless they address the basic financing and organizational issues that drive most service provision. This continues to be the case in a number of projects created under President Bush's New Freedom Initiative, seeking to remove barriers to community care for persons with disabilities.

One major initiative, introduced with great fanfare at the end of the Clinton administration, was the Ticket to Work and Work Incentives Improvement Act of 1999. The idea of having a voucher that an enrollee could give to any eligible provider sounded great to advocates who felt that the vocational rehabilitation system didn't serve them well. The idea itself was energized by a market philosophy that promotes competition and choice. As a member of a committee that recommended the concept to the House Ways and Means Committee,[15] I was skeptical that providers would risk engaging in a marketplace that tied payment closely to success in rehabilitation when success was highly uncertain. Despite much rhetoric and publicity, Ticket to Work has been used by very few clients, and the program thus far is a failure. Many in Washington have already given up on the concept, although the hype continues.

Bush's New Freedom Initiative continues with modest funding to expand consumers' control over their own services, such as those that allow clients to hire, fire, train, and supervise personal assistance attendants. The underlying values are very popular in the disability community, but many of the administrative and financial details of having clients or their designates manage their own services remain unclear. The potential problems of misuse of funds, life-threatening gaps in care, poor-quality care, and much more suggest that we should be careful to avoid confusing appealing rhetoric with reality. Based on the statements of Washington policy makers and the press, one might think that all Americans have superb information-seeking and decision-making skills and can negotiate through our convoluted health and long-term-care systems. Some obviously do. But one need do no more than peruse the studies of health literacy and what people actually understand about the programs in which they are enrollees to become a skeptic.[16] The difficulty faced by Medicare enrollees in choosing drug plans under the new Part D Medicare Program attests to this problem. Nevertheless, it is essential to remember the importance of individual control over one's circumstances, and the value of respecting individual preferences. But we have to make sure that our interventions fit reality.

Nursing homes remain the big item in the long-term-care picture, with about 1.44 million patients in these institutions in 2004. Surprisingly, the nursing home population has not grown as expected as the population ages, and occupancy rates have gone down, perhaps in part because of advances in delaying disabilities and new home and community alternatives.[17] It is important to note, however, that when patients become substantially incapacitated with many impairments in daily living and cognitive decline, the nursing home may be the best alternative for meaningfully organizing the assistance they need on a continuing basis, and the most economically feasible way of providing these services.

Most nursing homes are private, either small entrepreneurial enterprises or part of large national chains. There are good nursing homes that provide sophisticated and compassionate care responsive to the social and medical needs of their clients, but care in many institutions remains variable and in others it is highly deficient. Poor quality in nursing homes has been a continuing concern in Congress. Following an important Institute of Medicine study in 1986,[18] improvements were made, including reducing what had been the common use of patient restraints and the excessive use of psychoactive drugs to sedate patients. The Omnibus Budget Reconciliation Act of 1987 (OBRA-87) mandated a number of new standards and enforcement methods, including a comprehensive survey evaluation of patients' problems and needed services at admission, at least yearly, and whenever patients' status significantly changed. At the time, as a member of the U.S. Advisory Committee on Vital and Health Statistics, I was involved in helping to design the new nursing home evaluation. It was a difficult task that involved many people and numerous technical challenges, but the result has helped make the status of nursing home patients more transparent.

Nevertheless, many quality problems remain, and enforcement is weak. Government regulation focuses more on such issues as facility safety than on more difficult, but probably more important, quality issues. Safety and quality are not always the same. Maintaining function requires that patients be kept active and ambulatory to the extent possible, but ambulatory patients have more falls and accidents than patients who are sedated in bed. In any case, government has limited leverage in many instances, since providers are not competing vigorously for the most incapacitated clients, nor, given the reimbursement rates typically provided, do they have the sophisticated staff needed to provide complicated care. Although nursing home violations are now posted on the CMS web site for all to see, it is not clear that this information has any real practical import.

Reimbursement is a key aspect affecting care as states, facing budgetary difficulties, attempt to ratchet down reimbursement rates. Many nursing home patients require very intensive services, but the number of staff available inevitably depends on reimbursement. Such staffing importantly influences quality. The Boren Amendment in 1980 uplifted the nursing home industry by requiring that reimbursements be "reasonable and adequate to meet the costs which must be incurred by efficiently and economically operated facilities in order to provide care and services in conformity with applicable state and federal laws, regulations, and quality and safety standards."[19] Most states kept their budgets constrained by underpaying providers and cutting corners. Generally, the states that paid their providers better had programs with the most limited scope and eligibility. So, for many states, it has been a trade-off between serving more people or paying providers more. States protested against the Boren Amendment, seeing it as a threat to the financial viability of their Medicaid programs, state budget integrity, and administrative authority; it was repealed in 1997.[20]

Nursing homes that depend almost exclusively on Medicaid reimbursement, making cost shifting from more generous payers less possible, are especially disadvantaged. Approximately 15 percent of nursing homes are predominantly Medicaid; they are concentrated in the poorest regions of the country and serve the most disadvantaged clients, who are disproportionately members of minority groups. These institutions have far fewer nurses and other personnel, and many health-related deficiencies.[21] If we seriously regulated them on the basis of quality, they would be candidates for closure, but the alternatives are unclear, and the options available to their clients are very limited. The repeal of the Boren Amendment exacerbated the problem, but as Vincent Mor and his colleagues have noted, we need new policy initiatives that take better account of unmet need and of how to serve these clients more appropriately. Among the options they propose are an interventionist approach to increase funding for these deprived facilities, better training for nursing home managers, public takeover of failing facilities, and protections for displaced clients when institutions fail. [22]

A major issue in most nursing homes involves the training, supervision, skills, and capacities of nursing home personnel. The larger, more professionalized and sophisticated nursing homes may have the entire array of professional expertise, including physical therapy, nutrition, rehabilitation, social work, pain management, recreational and activities support, and much more; others have very little. Even walking through some of the more highly evaluated nursing homes, one is impressed by the large numbers of patients passively lined up in wheelchairs in the halls, seemingly vegetating and neglected, their plaintive pleas ignored by busy staff rushing by. Whenever I see this, it reminds me of my professional experiences decades ago in the large public custodial mental hospitals. This institutional custodial appearance is in major contrast to some of the teaching nursing homes I have visited, which convey an entirely different climate of activity, engagement, and compassion.

State and federal minimum requirements for staffing are modest, and nursing homes generally meet or exceed them but fall short of standards recommended by informed professional groups. The problems extend beyond numbers, however. Most personal care is provided by nursing aides who are poorly paid and have little training and high turnover. Many are kind, caring, compassionate people and develop loving relationships with patients. Others, feeling harassed and put upon, may neglect and abuse patients. As has been true in most large and inadequately staffed institutions, major direct-care responsibilities are given to those with the least training and lowest pay (and often no health insurance), who themselves face economic and social adversities. Nursing homes are not viewed as good places to work; they have difficulty attracting the best nurses or other personnel and are not of much interest to physicians either. Moreover, most members of these professions have received little preparation in dealing thoughtfully with nursing home residents. Appropriate supervision of those who provide the most direct personal services is often lacking, and highly disabled, dependent elderly, especially those without loved ones who visit frequently, are often at the mercy of these service workers.

One major challenge is to bring better-trained and skillful personnel to these institutions and programs. Physicians have only a limited role in nursing home care, and the quality of care depends primarily on motivated and well-prepared nurses. Until recently, however, nursing schools did little to provide their students in geriatrics and gerontology with special skills to provide excellent care to elderly people. With support from the John A. Hartford Foundation, an Institute for Geriatric Nursing was established at New York University to improve health care of older adults. The Institute took as its charge to bring geriatric nursing to nursing education throughout the country, thereby improving nursing practice in nursing homes, stimulating new research and policy initiatives, and developing nursing leadership in geriatrics. The charge is large and the course is difficult, particularly in view of the many financial, cultural, and institutional barriers facing nursing homes and long-term care. I have been privileged to serve on the Institute's National Board of Advisors and to watch how much thoughtful, motivated, and highly skillful leaders can accomplish. This is a very small piece of a much larger challenge, and it will take many such efforts to change the culture and practice of long-term care.[23]

We are increasingly able to understand and evaluate patterns of care and deficiencies in quality in nursing homes, and we are beginning to encourage higher practice standards. Nursing homes are contained institutions that, despite all their problems, make it possible to identify needs, train personnel, and supervise performance. But, as already noted, few elderly want to end up in nursing homes, and increasingly we are developing a range of community alternatives, such as home care and foster care. Services are more dispersed in the community and much more difficult to monitor and supervise. We must understand that maintaining patients in community programs does not ensure that they receive the services or professional quality they need. It is even easier to get lost and neglected in the community than in an institution, where care patterns may be more visible. As we continue to develop a menu of community care options, we must think carefully about the manner in which we can reasonably supervise personnel, monitor quality, and provide needed correctives.

There will always remain a need for nursing homes or comparable institutions. The challenge is to avoid the inevitable tendency for these institutions to take on a custodial character, to make patients more passive and dependent than they need be, and to undermine respect and a sense of dignity. The tasks are difficult and even among the best institutions one sees such inclinations. There is a growing consensus that the culture of nursing homes requires change, but culture change is a formidable task and difficult to sustain. There are important efforts underway that capture the imagination of many people involved in these institutions. The Eden Alternative, a philosophy introduced by Dr. William Thomas, a nursing home physician in New York State, has wide appeal; in its own words, it seeks "to create coalitions of people and organizations that are committed to creating better social and physical environments for people . . . helping others create enlivening environments and the elimination of the plagues of Loneliness, Helplessness, and Boredom."[24] Among its basic principles are "to place maximum possible decision-making authority into the hands of the Elders or into the hands of those closest to them." Institutions following this philosophy seek to make the environment more homelike, introducing plants, animals, and children. There are no rigorous evaluations of the Eden approach, or for that matter any of the other such models, but there are indications that they can contribute to enhancing the quality of life of residents and staff.[25]

One derivation from the Eden Alternative is the Green House Project, also developed by Dr. William Thomas. Seeking to change the culture of long-term care, Green House organizes houses of eight to ten people, blending with neighborhoods and using architecture and interior design to create warm living spaces while providing the support and assistance with activities of daily living that residents require.[26] Residents have private rooms and baths and access to all home facilities, without the institutional features we associate with nursing homes. The Green House focuses first on living situation and responsiveness to resident need, without making health care the central focus. It also seeks to transform staffing consistent with the ideals of the Eden Alternative. This movement on its face seems very attractive, but at this time it involves very few people. There are plans to develop Green Houses in a number of states, but the movement is just a fragment of a solution to a very large problem. There are important questions relating to its effects on quality of care and on health, its affordability under existing funding structures, and how expansion can be financed. Rosalie Kane, a distinguished long-term-care researcher at the University of Minnesota, is doing an evaluation study of one such project in Tupelo, Mississippi, and has observed many positive reactions to living and working in the Green House.[27] The tough questions at this point still remain to be answered, although optimists view it as a positive example of what it is possible to do in changing the culture of nursing homes.

Another model involves eleven not-for-profit nursing homes in Wisconsin under the rubric of the Wellspring Alliance. This approach seeks to improve the clinical care provided to clients while also creating a better environment by empowering employees with the skills needed to do their jobs better and have more of a voice in goal attainment. Here the means include consultation and education by a geriatric nurse practitioner, shared training, the use of inter-disciplinary resource teams to develop appropriate interventions, and sharing comparative outcome data on clients. A fifteen-month qualitative evaluation of the model by sophisticated assessors concluded that there were many positive results.[28]

Long-term care is a large and decentralized area built around relatively small institutions and programs, and one sees many efforts at innovation. Sustaining culture change over time and maintaining enthusiasm and momentum are no small matters, and exceedingly difficult. Change is more sustainable when the structure of reimbursement and regulation is supportive and not obstructive of efforts to improve quality. We need a wide range of alternatives to fit people's varied life situations, preferences, and levels of incapacity. In the final analysis, we must remember that long-term-care clients are in many respects among our most vulnerable, and we cannot depend on wishful thinking. We must have the information that assures us that clients are receiving appropriate clinical and social care. If we have learned anything from the history of deinstitutionalization in other areas over the past fifty years, we should know that many of the terrible things that can happen to people in institutions can also happen to people in community settings, including their own homes, foster care, and assisted living facilities. There are many constructive and innovative endeavors underway in long-term care, but continuing vigilance and requiring increased accountability for providing quality care would be prudent policy.

Part II

The Struggle for Solutions

There is much consensus that major changes are required in our health care system, but there is also a great deal of disagreement about the way forward. Many interests seek to protect their own turf, and faced with actual choices for change, they often prefer the status quo, however deficient, to uncertainty and the prospect of losing ground. Achieving significant changes will require defining a broad middle ground where enough of the players see themselves as having something to gain.

Everyone wants more quality unless they feel their ox is being gored. Thus, introducing and implementing quality systems requires getting the incentives right, developing broad coalitions and alliances, helping individuals and groups overcome their fears and insecurities, and making people more comfortable with a climate of change. To achieve these goals we have to avoid the blame game and help professionals and groups improve their performance in ways that build their confidence and self-respect. No one aspires to be a low-quality provider, and we don't improve performance by insults or stigma.

We also have to face the problem of constraints realistically and learn to allocate our talents and resources more wisely. American health care is a rich system, the envy of the world from a resource point of view. But even we have to have constraints, especially if we are to meet our common aspiration to see that everyone has access to needed care. Constraints are connected to quality, because quality is often enhanced by doing less and by focusing on doing what we know is effective and worthwhile. But there is much disagreement on what is worth doing, and we need processes in place to ensure that our decisions are thoughtful and fair, open to modification with new information and evidence, and seen as legitimate by patients and the public.

Both enhancing quality and imposing realistic constraints require that the public and patients trust the health care system. While patients still trust their personal doctors, there is much distrust of the health system and health leaders. This has alarmed many professionals and professional groups, and they are struggling with ways to demonstrate their trustworthiness to the public. We have to build on these efforts, working with organizations in the public and private sectors, with media, and with the general public. With more trust we will have a better opportunity to arrive at necessary compromises, and take the steps required to build quality systems and allocate care fairly.

Chapter 7

The Quest for Quality

Repeated studies going back over decades demonstrate that the quality of health care falls far short of what could be achieved. Medicine is a complex and ever-changing endeavor, and it is inevitable that there will always be significant gaps between what is theoretically possible and the actual provision of care in numerous settings, involving hundreds of millions of transactions. One need not think in utopian terms, however, to understand the magnitude of deficiencies and the mortality, illness, and disability that are avoidable even in a very imperfect system. Observations of avoidable errors in care have been enumerated over many decades, but in recent years there have been more serious efforts to build and disseminate the evidence to help guide appropriate clinical decision making. Evidence-based medicine constitutes an important element of the quality movement

Evidence-based medicine seeks to inform practice by upgrading clinical knowledge through systematic review and synthesis of results from randomized controlled clinical trials. David Sackett, the physician who popularized the evidence-based concept, and his colleagues define it "as the conscientious, explicit, and judicious use of current best evidence in making decisions about the care of individual patients."[1] Such evidence-based medicine is seen as the source for developing evidence-based guidelines. The effort to draw systematically upon the best research is essential, but much in medicine remains uncertain or unknown, and much remains in dispute. Moreover, quality of care involves factors well beyond the actions of individual physicians.

It is not in dispute that we pay a high price for failing to remedy serious and modifiable quality problems. Many medical errors are due to poor system design, outmoded technologies, poor supervision, dysfunctional teams, lack of communication and coordination, and unclear procedures and expectations. The Institute of Medicine's (IOM) estimate that between forty-four thousand and ninety-eight thousand deaths and hundreds of thousands of injuries each year are due to medical error has been widely disseminated.[2] Some experts who work in the medical-error field believe this range to be an underestimate, while others see it as inflated. Nevertheless, there is no disagreement that we have a profound problem that requires major interventions. Since the first IOM report in 2000, many corrective efforts have gone forward, but progress has been slow.[3] It is difficult to change complex systems and the cultures and values they embody and get individuals to modify habitual work patterns. Improving quality of care is a multidimensional challenge that involves technology, economic incentives, organizational coordination, and individual behavior-change strategies.

At the individual level of evidence-based care, there has been much research over the years documenting gaps in providing medical care of quality. An extensive review of the literature in 1998 by RAND Corporation researchers found that only half the population received recommended preventive care, 70 percent recommended acute care, and 60 percent recommended chronic care. They also found that studies reported much care that was not appropriate.[4] This led to an ambitious RAND effort, published in the *New England Journal of Medicine* in 2003, that reported on 439 quality-of-care indicators applied to a large national sample.[5] Using interview responses and medical record reviews, the investigators assessed the extent to which these respondents received appropriate and inappropriate care.

Overall, the study found that 55 percent of participants received the care that would have been recommended by medical panels that reviewed the medical literature and national guidelines. The study did not find large differences in the failures to provide appropriate preventive, acute, and chronic care; in each case almost half the patients did not receive recommended services. There appeared to be large variations among medical conditions, with especially poor care in the case of alcohol dependence, hip fracture, atrial fibrillation, dyspepsia, and ulcer disease, and comparably good quality in the treatment of senile cataract, breast cancer, and prenatal care. Although the investigators reported more problems with underprovision of care than with inappropriate provision, the study was not designed to address inappropriate care, and most of the 439 quality indicators studied were focused on underprovision. One can dispute many particular aspects of this ambitious study, but it would be difficult to disagree with the authors' understated conclusion that "the gap between what we know works and what is actually done is substantial enough to warrant attention."[6]

What Accounts for the Care Provided?

It has long been recognized that the supply of doctors, specialists, and health facilities, and the ways institutions and professionals are paid, affect the amounts and types of services provided. A half-century ago, Milton Roemer,[7] a public health professor at UCLA, noted that the rate of hospital admission in varying geographic areas was closely related to the number of hospital beds in these areas, a phenomenon referred to as Roemer's Law. In 1970 John Bunker,[8] an anesthesiologist and health services researcher, documented the close association between the number of surgeons in a locality and the amount of surgery performed. Both economic incentives and the fact that professionals do what they are trained to do, explain these patterns.

In 1973 John Wennberg and Alan Gittelsohn[9] published a classic paper in *Science* on small area variations in health care delivery in thirteen hospital service areas in Vermont. They found large differences in resource investments, expenditures, and utilization of care among neighboring communities that could not be reasonably accounted for by differences in illness. Ironically, Wennberg later explained in an interview that the paper was published in *Science* (one of the premier journals in the world) because the major medical journals would not publish it.[10] We now have a large body of research in the United States and around the world continuing to document the same types of variations in many areas of health care.[11] Among the important conclusions are that variations in utilization are related to the availability of physicians, specialists, and hospital beds, as well as insurance coverage; the magnitude of variations increases with greater uncertainty and for procedures that are more discretionary; there is no clear relationship between appropriate care and high and low rates of utilization; and higher rates of utilization and expenditures are not usually associated with better outcomes and are sometimes associated with poorer ones.[12] It seems likely that the culture of physicians in particular localities and hospitals and the practice norms that they come to share play some part, but understanding how these influences occur and why is still mostly guesswork. The research literature observes deficiencies of both under- and overprovision, but many questions persist about what the proper standards of care should be to achieve the most cost-effective outcomes.

Some Issues in Evidence-Based Practice

Evidence-based medicine and its implementation through practice guidelines represent a significant trend that promises to bring greater clarity and rationality to the practice of medicine. Impressive advances in implementation have been made in large care programs such as Kaiser Permanente and the Veterans Affairs health system that have the size, administrative structures, and managerial capacity that allow investment in information systems, electronic clinical records, appropriate prompts and reminders, and feedback to help physicians improve their performance. Of course, much uncertainty remains in medical decision making, and it is important to protect physicians' discretion to override practice guidelines when they believe the clinical situation requires it. Evidence-based medicine and practice guidelines are based on average experience overall, but there is much variation among patients' health situations and responses to treatment. Thus, protecting physician discretion, as Kaiser-Permanente proudly announces as its policy, is prudent. But physicians should be accountable for providing credible justification for their decisions when they override evidence-based guidelines.

For many reasons, treatment plans for any individual patient may vary from recommendations that are based solely on the results of randomized clinical trials. Most trials of treatment efficacy occur under highly controlled situations with patients who typically have no complicating comorbidities and who usually are not representative of the gender, age, and race distributions of the population. The average efficacy observed in clinical trials may not equally apply to all segments of the population, but study subgroups are often too small to make reliable estimates for them. What makes sense over an entire population may have less validity for any particular patient. In usual practice, patients typically have many comorbidities that complicate treatment, and such comorbidities increase with age.[13] Patients, depending on age, gender, ethnicity, or comorbidities, may respond differently to treatment, and have different preferences about the trade-offs involved in their care. Evidence-based practice should instruct and help guide treatment, but doctors must remain sensitive to the complexities and uncertainties of scientific knowledge and patients' individual circumstances.

A few examples help illustrate the issues. There is increasing enthusiasm for the use of statins to reduce risk for coronary heart disease among persons with high cholesterol. The evidence for prevention among younger men at high risk is persuasive. These drugs are marketed aggressively, and the findings in studies of young and middle-aged men are commonly generalized to the entire population. In the case of younger women, however, the evidence is less persuasive, and there is little evidence to support statin treatment for the elderly. John Abramson, a member of the clinical faculty at the Harvard Medical School, concludes, after analyzing the supporting evidence for the treatment guidelines for cholesterol, that they "fail miserably."[14]

Similarly, there are significant gender differences in physiological response in cardiovascular[15] and other areas. Women also metabolize some drugs differently than men,[16] and drugs may have different effects, as was shown in the findings on effects of aspirin in the Woman's Health Study.[17]

The treatment of heart failure in black and white populations provides a different kind of example. Prior data suggested that treatment with isosorbide dinitrate and hyzdralazine (a branded medication called BiDil) had no benefit for white patients with heart failure but seemed to enhance survival among black patients. A randomized clinical trial with black patients found this treatment reduced mortality by 43 percent.[18] The use of skin color here is a crude proxy for other unrecognized differences, and use of race as a basis of treatment raises controversial issues, since the race category itself is ambiguous and commonly misused.[19] But this and other research indicates that there are important subgroup differences in how people respond to treatment by age, gender, race, as well as other morbidities. Marketing efforts to promote drugs, treatments, and even practice guidelines often gloss over these differences.

Comorbid diseases, frequent among the elderly, pose serious problems for the use of commonly available practice guidelines. Almost half of persons over age 65 have three or more chronic conditions, and approximately one-fifth have five or more. Medicare enrollees with five or more conditions account for about two-thirds of Medicare expenditures.[20] One study sought to assess the applicability of commonly used practice guidelines for the elderly who had a number of comorbid conditions.[21] The researchers developed a hypothetical scenario involving treatment of a seventy-nine-year-old woman with five chronic diseases, all of moderate severity (osteoporosis, osteoarthritis, type 2 diabetes mellitus, hypertension, and chronic obstructive pulmonary disease). Applying the guidelines resulted in a medical regimen with many medications, potential adverse drug interactions, and treatment-induced negative outcomes. They also report that following such recommended regimens would in all likelihood be an unsustainable treatment burden for the patient, involving serious difficulties in adherence and self-management. In the example studied, the patient would have received twelve medications, required complicated follow-up care, and had medication costs conservatively estimated at $406 per month. The authors express concern that simplistic pay-for-performance programs could provide disincentives for treating such patients and when treating them could provide inducements for poor management. This is an issue that requires serious attention.

As noted earlier, many organizations are producing practice guidelines, often seeking to promote their own economic or professional interests. The typical practicing physician may receive numerous guidelines recommending different ways of treating the same condition, and it is difficult to determine which one most accurately represents the evidence. Large organizations like Kaiser Permanente, Veterans Affairs, and the English National Health Service can make their own informed judgments, but the average physician has no comparable guidance. The federal government, through its Agency for Health-care Research and Quality, initially did outstanding work in this area, but the backlash from special interests required the agency to get out of the guideline business.

A major difficulty in encouraging a more evidence-based practice system is our pluralistic plans and provider organizations and the prevalence of many small practices that lack the infrastructure or direction to take advantage of new technological possibilities and compilation of scientific information. Because physicians commonly deal with numerous insurers, in most instances no insurer is sufficiently dominant within their practices to significantly alter behavior. Some insurers are developing quality initiatives, including pay for performance systems, but typically insurers lack sufficient market penetration to significantly alter individual physicians' practices. From the typical physician's perspective, the incentives are too small, and the effort and economic and learning costs associated with changing seem too large. In their frustration, they justify their inaction by denigrating practice guidelines as "cookbook medicine." Stronger incentives rather than more exhortation are required to stimulate the needed practice changes.

Paying for Performance

It has always been understood that payment can be a powerful incentive and that it affects how institutions and professionals work, but it is difficult to design such incentives so they are not subverted. The Medicare hospital prospective payment system (PPS), for example, induced hospitals to work more efficiently and reduce length of stay. PPS also induced hospitals to code diagnoses to maximize reimbursement and to transfer patients to nursing homes for some of their care in order to reduce the costs of hospital care. Since the nursing homes were reimbursed as separate facilities, some hospitals converted some of their beds to nursing home beds to increase overall payment.

Increasingly, health plans are coming to the conclusion that one way of improving quality is to reward doctors for achieving important specified patient outcomes. However, unlike large, organized systems, many doctors have too few patients from any single health plan for these incentives to have a significant effect on their overall remuneration. Nevertheless, a number of health plans are devising payment incentives to reward quality outcomes, and in some instances plans are cooperating to promote and reward common quality objectives.[22]

Although the idea of paying for performance sounds simple enough, there are many complexities.[23] If the goal is to bring medical practice overall to high levels of performance, we need fair incentives that reward both high-quality performers and those who improve. If our incentive system measures quality in terms of disease outcomes and patient adherence and satisfaction, any reasonable system must take account of differences in the vulnerabilities, attitudes, and behavior of varying populations. This requires sophisticated case mix adjustment, a technique that remains underdeveloped. Moreover, medicine is highly complex; it involves many diseases and treatments and trade-offs in care, and any good incentive system seeks overall quality improvement and not only on the indicators being measured. Thus, the measures must be clear enough to communicate goals, but not so simple that they can easily be gamed. There are approaches for managing some of these issues, but they are complex and largely untested. In short, pay-for-performance is a work in progress, and its ultimate success remains unknown. Since no specified system of incentives can deal comprehensively with the complexity and dynamic nature of medical care, we must continue to seek ways to induce greater professionalism and aspirations for excellence.

Promoting Improved Quality in the NHS

One of the most ambitious efforts, first introduced in the UK's NHS in 2004, sought to significantly upgrade quality of care in general practice and reward doctors who take on added care responsibilities.[24] The NHS has advantages, compared with the United States, in that it is a unified service involving all patients, and NHS doctors are not faced with the competing and conflicting incentives characteristic of our pluralistic system. Another advantage is that this initiative is being introduced at a time when England has been substantially upgrading its investments in the NHS, and thus quality payments constitute a substantial added income increment constituting 18 percent of general practitioner (GP) remuneration.[25] In addition, the NHS has been investing significantly in enhancing primary care capacities, involving a one-third increase in funding over three years. The system being put in place covers a wide range of objectives and rewards doctors for incremental improvements as well as larger changes. Using a point system that goes to a maximum of 1,050 points, practices can be rewarded for a range of improvements including meeting clinical standards for a variety of important diseases, achieving organizational standards, including improved medical records and practice management, enhancing the experience of patients, and providing a number of additional services. Rewarding practice performance rather than only the work of individual clinicians is believed to encourage collaboration and teamwork. It is too early to assess how this system actually works in practice, but it is thoughtfully designed, had initial strong doctor support (GPs voted overwhelmingly to approve the contract), and the process of implementation and the results are clearly worth watching. The experience cannot be generalized easily to the very different American context but we can learn from how the incentives are designed, monitored, and impact practice.

New Medicare Initiatives

In the United States, Medicare is the "big guy" on the block and has the market potential to promote quality efforts. The Centers for Medicare and Medicaid Services (CMS), which administers the program, is a much-watched, often-maligned federal agency and faces many political influences from the White House, Congress, and other groups. While CMS potentially carries a big stick, it moves cautiously, seeking broad consultation and partnerships. Large demonstration projects precede broader implementation. In 2003, CMS launched the Hospital Quality Incentive Demonstration Project to see if financial incentives could improve quality of inpatient care in five clinical areas: acute myocardial infarction; coronary artery bypass surgery; heart failure; community-acquired pneumonia; and hip and knee replacement. Each participating hospital received a composite quality score. Hospitals performing in the top decile received a bonus of 2 percent of DRG payments for the measured condition; those in the second decile received a 1 percent bonus. While providing bonuses for high-performing hospitals, the demonstration does not penalize poor performers.

In November 2005, CMS issued a press release reporting that results, after the first year, showed that hospitals participating in the quality incentive program had measurable improvements in care. CMS reported that quality improved in all five clinical areas measured, with average improvement of 6.6 percent over thirty-three quality indicators relevant to these conditions. CMS provided bonuses of almost nine million dollars to hospitals that improved most. These results are encouraging, but this report does not inform us about changes that would be occurring in any case given the attention now focused on hospital quality issues. A curious fact reported by CMS is that scores of the poorest-performing hospitals, which received no bonuses, improved the most. This encourages skepticism that the changes are really due to the pay-for-performance incentives.

In 2004, CMS initiated a Doctor's Office Quality Project that sought to improve quality of care and assess the feasibility of defined measurement components using various data sources. The project focused on clinical measures of care for coronary artery disease, diabetes, heart failure, hypertension, osteoarthritis, and preventive care. A second aspect included patients' experience with care, including access, continuity, communication, health promotion, and other measures, adapted from the extensive work done on the Consumer Assessment of Health Plans Surveys (CAHPS™).[26] This effort, sponsored by the Agency for Healthcare Research and Quality, measures consumer experience with doctors and specialists, access to care, physician communication, customer service, claims processing, and related concerns. A third element of the project collects data from office staffs about clinical information systems, patient education support, and care management. The purpose is to develop systems that allow useful feedback to doctors to help them improve their work. CMS also has a variety of other efforts such as one that helps physicians in smaller practices to develop electronic clinical records and improve their information technology.

In 2003 the Medicare Prescription Drug, Improvement and Modernization Act established two new performance-based contracting projects. The Voluntary Chronic Care Improvement Program focuses on patients with conditions like congestive heart failure, diabetes, and chronic obstructive pulmonary disease; it enlists experienced organizations to help enrollees manage their health by means that include guidance for self-care and physician technical support to manage clinical information about the patient. Participating organizations such as disease-management organizations, insurers, physician group practices, and the like are expected to meet performance standards for clinical quality, patient satisfaction, and cost savings and are to refund payments if they underperform. A Care Management Performance Pilot Program will pay physicians to treat chronic conditions using health information technology (such as patient e-mail and clinical alerts) and evidence-based criteria. Physicians who meet performance standards will be paid on a per-enrollee basis. A major limitation of this initiative is the requirement of budget neutrality, which may not be fully realistic given the uncertainty of the assumption that quality improvement efforts reduce costs.

A large number of private-sector organizations are seeking to stimulate improvements in the quality of care and organizational collaborations toward common goals.[27] Involved participants include accreditation agencies, business groups, quality-assurance organizations, public interest groups, health think tanks, foundations, large health plans, and professional organizations. There are hundreds of these organizations, but no one really exercises sufficient leverage or authority to implement broad change. CMS, of course, theoretically has the leverage, but it is politically constrained by the many interests that have a stake in its decisions. There is much innovation and creativity in the system, but little capacity for systematic implementation. Compared with current efforts in the National Health Service in the UK, we lack the centralized command-and-control structure to require uniform changes, and unlike the UK, which is substantially increasing its health care funding, we are carrying out new initiatives in a context of budget neutrality and a desire to reduce increases in health care costs. While we are the most luxuriously funded system in the world, it is far more difficult to redistribute than to use additional funding as an incentive for change.

The pay-for-performance efforts now being introduced face additional difficulties. CMS's Hospital Quality Incentive approach, for example, seeks to reward the two top deciles in the hope that the incentive will stimulate a broader quest for excellence. But the majority of hospitals have little chance to be rewarded, and these may be the institutions that most require our concerted efforts. We risk rewarding the already privileged segments of our health system. Also, the demonstrations, for obvious reasons, enlist volunteers, but volunteers are always different in many ways from the overall population, and the interventions that are successful in changing these organizations and clinicians may not be generalizable.

Attuning Patients to Quality

Many health reformers aim to encourage patients to make health care choices on the basis of quality as well as price. In recent years much effort has been applied to measuring quality in health plans, hospitals, and other settings so that purchasers and patients could be better prepared to make thoughtful choices. Some nonprofit organizations have developed ways of gathering and reporting health performance data that have served as prototypes. An early effort by the National Committee for Quality Assurance (NCQA) developed a Health Plan Data and Information Set (HEDIS) that has gone through a number of iterations and expansions and is used in accreditation evaluations, by regulatory agencies, and in other private and public initiatives. The HEDIS measures are informative but limited to a relatively small number of process measures that have relied mostly on voluntary and unstandardized reporting by health plans. Plans that are performing poorly could withhold their data from public view; thus, the information available to the public is biased. In the long run, the value of HEDIS may be less in the sophistication of the measures and the quality of reported performance data, and more in establishing a precedent for measuring comparative performance and making such information available to prospective purchasers.

Reliable quality assessment faces many technical challenges, and it is still very early in its evolution, but progress is being made in some important areas, such as cardiovascular surgery.[28] The process of evaluation itself and the dissemination of such information are incentives for improving care but they also have the potential downside of encouraging doctors and facilities to avoid high-risk patients. As noted earlier, efforts are underway to link evidence of good performance with increased financial payments. These efforts involve both technical and philosophical issues, but it is early in their evolution and we have much to learn about how such incentives work and their unintended consequences.[29]

Surveys indicate that while the public says they value this kind of consumer information, and there is growing evidence of more people using the Internet to acquire health and treatment information, ratings of health plans and providers are still not commonly used. Most sources of such information, including the government, health plans, and the media are not much trusted; people continue to get their guidance from relatives, friends, and their personal physicians.[30] Inertia also continues because people are more inclined to value personal experience than impersonal sources of information. When asked if they would prefer a familiar hospital to one rated as superior by experts, a majority of respondents continue to choose the familiar hospital.[31] There may be good reasons for them to do so. Moreover, once persons are part of a network of providers, the referral trajectory in many ways becomes inevitable.

Consider the example in 2004 of President Bill Clinton and his bypass surgery. Clinton and his family are sophisticated, well-informed consumers, highly intelligent and extremely well connected. They are also affluent and would be welcomed to any health facility in the nation. Indeed, most health system administrators would salivate over the publicity value of the public knowing that Bill Clinton went to their hospital for his care. Given where he lives, and where he was initially treated, Clinton would most naturally be referred to physicians at Columbia University Medical Center, an institution with a distinguished research reputation, and it is where he was eventually treated.

New York State has been a national leader in monitoring cardiovascular surgery and providing to the public data on hospital and surgical mortality rates associated with this procedure, adjusted for various possible biases. Theoretically, sophisticated medical consumers would seek care at hospitals with the lowest adjusted mortality for this procedure and for their chosen surgeon, but the latest data published on the Internet from the Department of Health indicated that Clinton's hospital had relatively high mortality for this surgery compared with other New York hospitals.[32] If one took these data seriously, one would seek to have surgery at a hospital with lower cardiovascular mortality. We don't know what Clinton's other considerations were in choosing care, and perhaps he made a wise choice. Perhaps he trusted his doctors' advice that the Columbia University Medical Center was the right place for him and perhaps he will someday tell us. What this anecdote indicates, however, is the magnitude of the challenge in creating structures where quality information actually drives individual choice.

Pay-for-performance programs focus on many of the most important, common, and costly illnesses. It remains unclear whether such efforts then draw attention away from other important areas where care is challenging. Care not measured, and thus not rewarded, may be neglected. For example, the quality measures for mental health and social care in the NHS general practice quality program are very limited and clearly inadequate. Does this mean, then, that these historically neglected areas will suffer even more neglect? There are hundreds of important things to do well in caring for patients. As people in education learned over and over again, you can provide incentives that lead schools to teach to the test, but this does not necessarily lead to the best education.

Barriers to Implementation

Physicians are often described as highly resistant to change, but the rapid adoption of new diagnostic and treatment approaches and technologies belie such easy characterization. Barriers to change include the need to choose among competing programs and systems, high start-up costs in many instances, the need to learn new systems and practice routines, inevitable inefficiencies that occur in new learning and transition phases, and threats to income. Even physicians who have adapted to new IT and other technologies and are enthusiastic about them attest to the commitment and hard work needed to make the transition. Compounding the challenges are the many uncertainties of a rapidly changing political and economic context, growing expectations and demands from all quarters, and an increasing sense of constrained time and reduced autonomy in a medical system that seems beset with problems and in disarray.

Much focus has been placed on consumerism and consumer information and choice, but questions remain about how much this emphasis can achieve. Progress has been made and continues to be made in developing information about performance. Measures of health plan performance as in HEDIS, CAHPS™, Picker Institute studies of patient experiences, and health plan surveys are all informative and useful, but they have not had the marketplace influence that advocates hoped. Employers and employees remain focused on costs, and, if anything, such focus is increasing as medical care costs escalate. Moreover, the types of information patients most want is difficult to provide in any reliable way. Patients most want information on specific doctors' technical competence, interpersonal skills, and caring, but as anyone knows who has examined the Web sites about physicians, this information isn't available. Hospital performance data are based on larger samples and are more statistically valid, but ambiguities remain about whether different hospitals' mix of patients is adequately taken into account so that the data are truly comparable. Moreover, knowing the overall hospital or HMO experience may tell little about one's chosen physician.

As I repeatedly note, and it can't be overstated, the key to quality improvement is the implementation of an electronic medical record, the ability of systems to communicate, the capacity to identify high-risk situations and take preventive action, and the use of well-organized feedback to provide information about best practices, alerts, and opportunities to assess and correct performance. Many vendors offer a bewildering variety of informational systems and disease-management programs. Understanding and choosing wisely among them is challenging. CMS has a program to help physicians in small- to medium-sized practices adopt high-quality information technology, but it refuses, for understandable reasons, to endorse any particular vendor product or service, and this is often the kind of assistance doctors most need as they confront bewildering choices. Research on choice suggests that while people want choices, too many choices become bewildering, leading individuals to opt out.[33]

Some of the large health systems that have successfully implemented sophisticated informational technology have invested impressive funds, expertise, and time in making these systems operational, retraining physicians and support personnel, keeping information up-to-date, expeditiously troubleshooting and correcting problems, and dealing with the natural reluctance among many participants to deal with the uncertainties of needed change. The challenges and anxieties faced by smaller practices are substantial, and good strategies to deal with them are yet to be developed.

Effective pay for performance must also support the goal of reinvigorating medical professionalism. Many observers, impatient to see change, have become cynical about professionalism and see calls for professionalism as self-serving. But most physicians care about quality, and their involvement and cooperation are essential in achieving the needed improvements. Physicians understand that the corpus of medical knowledge is large, and growing, and the human capacity to process and retain this information and use it wisely are limited. Physicians have much to gain by intelligent systems that inform and alert them and bring new knowledge to their attention. But discretion to use their judgment in individual situations must also be protected, and measuring and rewarding performance with a limited set of indicators that may not reflect the entire array of skills, practices, and judgments necessary may be inconsistent with the self-reflection, continued learning, and capacities necessary for excellence.

Supporting Medical Professionalism

The ability to practice good medicine depends on context. The incentives, demands, and pressures of practice can make it difficult to practice in ideal ways. Much of medical practice is local and influenced by community practice patterns and norms. In the absence of comparative practice information and clear guides as to how well one is doing, it is natural to believe oneself at or above the norm. Credible information to the contrary can be a motivating influence among physicians committed to professional values.

Physicians often feel powerless to alter the societal forces that affect how they practice. In earlier eras, young physicians commonly established independent practices or small partnerships. They typically could take as much time as they needed with each patient, adapting by extending the hours spent in patient care. Some physicians continue to practice in this way, but changes in financing, organization, and technology have made such adaptations less satisfactory. Physicians typically now have careers within organizational settings and must participate in large health plans and larger groups to survive economically. In more organized settings, the office pace may be scheduled or set by managers or peers concerned about productivity. Payment typically reinforces a focus on technical procedures and less attention on communication and instruction.

An important lesson learned in behavior change research is that cognitive awareness and intention are not sufficient to elicit desired behaviors. Implementation is more likely when participants can see realistically ways to overcome constraints. Models are needed that will help physicians understand how they can successfully build important values about patient care and quality into their everyday practice routines, particularly in smaller group settings with limited managerial expertise of the type that large integrated health programs can call on. Many quality-improvement approaches are being evaluated, ranging from the innovative use of nurse practitioners, physician assistants, and teams to computerized technologies for managing diseases and avoiding errors.[34]

In the absence of good road maps, physicians will adapt by finding comfortable practice niches or developing shortcuts, but unguided adaptations may not adhere to the values of medical professionalism or follow scientific knowledge. Shortcuts aren't necessarily bad, but they have to be carefully developed, evaluated and taught.[35]

Many organizations concerned with health care are active in addressing issues around professional responsibility and quality, and many physicians are devoting energy to improving accountability.[36] Specialty and other physician organizations will need to cooperate with government, health plans, and patient groups to devise feasible approaches. Improving quality, thus, requires coordinated initiatives in many different areas. It is unrealistic in our pluralistic system to expect interested groups to push in the same direction, but getting even some to agree to align their objectives and approaches will help. In the private sector, for example, a number of large employers, including General Motors, General Electric, and the Pacific Business Group on Health, came together to form the LeapFrog Group, a cooperative venture to improve patient safety and customer value in health care. The mission is to use their combined purchasing power to encourage hospitals to introduce certain patient safety features, such as computer physician-order entry. Insurance plans seeking to change physician behavior by paying for performance are likely to be much more effective if they agree to encourage and reward the same practices, or at least agree not to work at cross-purposes. If they can cooperate successfully with medical specialty societies in setting objectives and encouraging change, such efforts will gain momentum and have a better chance to succeed. Developing consistent objectives, policies, and incentives is a challenging task, and implementation will remain messy and incomplete. But significant progress is possible if institutions, organizations, and participants work together in promoting shared goals.

Chapter 8

Setting Fair Limits

In 1998 the marketing of Viagra, the first effective sexual-enhancement drug, brought the issue of rationing, a topic widely discussed among health care experts for many years, to a larger public. There have always been well-understood limits on some procedures seen as having no clear medical purpose, such as many cosmetic surgery procedures, but the introduction of Viagra posed more difficult policy issues about payment for enhancement drugs. Viagra, whatever its lifestyle-enhancement value, had a serious medical purpose in treating men with erectile dysfunction (ED) associated with aging and such conditions as prostate cancer, diabetes, and cardiovascular disease. ED is self-reported, however, and the definition of adequate and normal sexual performance is itself highly subjective. Moreover, the prevalence of ED and the demand for Viagra were unclear but were expected to be large. The drug was a highly effective treatment and much superior to other known treatments for ED. By usual criteria, the drug should be covered by insurance, but policy makers worried about its lifestyle uses and costs and sought to find ways to restrict access. A simple way adopted by many insurers in the United States was to restrict the number of pills, such as one a week, but other countries made more efforts, in addition, to restrict access more closely to those who had a relevant medical condition. Whatever the reasons given, much of the motivation was simply economic, although complicated by notions of morality that have always played a big part in medical determinations.

Initially, there wasn't much political attention to Viagra. Senator Bob Dole, a prominent Republican politician who had run for president and who was a survivor of prostate cancer, promoted the drug in TV and other media advertisements. Increased attention was focused on Viagra and other new sexual-enhancement drugs following enactment of a new prescription Medicare benefit, and the increasing cost problems in the Medicaid program, which was spending a reported $38 million each year for such drugs. When New York City Comptroller Alan Hevesi reported that 198 offenders had received Viagra through New York's Medicaid program, an uproar ensued. In California, under pressure from the Bush administration, the governor ordered that state officials not provide ED drugs to any Medicaid enrollee who had been convicted of a sex crime.[1] And the controversy of who should get access continues.

Following passage of the new Medicare prescription drug benefit, CMS administrator Mark McClellan announced that under existing legislation he did not have the authority to exclude coverage of ED medications for elderly enrollees. In June 2005, the House of Representatives passed an amendment by a vote of 285-121 to disallow coverage of ED drugs such as Viagra, Cialis, and Levitra in Medicare and Medicaid.[2] Charles Grassley, chair of the Senate Finance Committee, said that if ED drugs were not restricted they could cost Medicare and Medicaid $2 billion over the next decade. Representative Steven King, a Republican from Iowa who sponsored the House legislation, complained that we are taxing young people "to subsidize Grandpa's recreational sex." He told the press that "sex is never medically necessary. If it was, priests wouldn't live into the 90s."[3]

In October 2005 Congress passed a bill that banned Medicare and Medicaid from covering erectile dysfunction medications and sent it to the president. Representative Nathan Deal from Georgia, who sponsored the bill in the House of Representatives, contended that it would save the federal government $690 million over five years. State Medicaid programs can continue to provide these drugs but would receive no federal matching funds. This provision was seen as offsetting renewal of other benefits for low-income beneficiaries.

The rationing of ED drugs around the world can be seen as an example of successful rationing, because restrictions have generally been proven to be politically feasible and for the most part acceptable to the public.[4] Governments have either excluded Viagra as a benefit or made it contingent on having a medical problem as assessed by a physician. As Rudolf Klein and Heidrun Sturm sagaciously observe, while it is difficult to differentiate medications seeking to improve function and quality of life from "lifestyle drugs," a reasonable working distinction is that "lifestyle drugs" are those "where the patient rather than the doctor not only diagnoses the condition but also can demand a specific remedy."[5] They note that many of the governments that instituted controls managed to steer a prudent financial course while being reasonably objective. Officials distinguished between needs defined by patient demand and those defined by doctors, showing respect for medical autonomy by leaving room for medical discretion. Viagra reveals many of the issues and tensions characteristic of rationing debates, but as the following discussion will show, Viagra constitutes a relatively easy case.

Types of Rationing

The term "rationing" has strong negative connotations in political discussion in the United States and is commonly used as a way to discredit medical initiatives that opponents dislike. There is broad understanding that we must have limits on what we spend on medical care if it is not to squeeze out equally important priorities. Whatever the many quiet ways we limit provision of care and costs, Americans seem unwilling to accept direct limitations. This important aspect of the managed care backlash and the retreat among health insurers trying to restrain cost has contributed to resumption of the cost spiral. People seem to be more willing to accept impediments to access when they see these impediments as just the way things are. Thus, waiting for appointments, waiting in a doctor's office, travel distance, short consultations with revisits, and much more are seen as the nature of everyday life, not as ways of controlling or limiting consumption.

Klein and his colleagues have elucidated at least seven types of rationing, many of which would not necessarily be viewed as rationing.[6] Among them are rationing by denial, as perhaps represented by the limitations on service for people without health insurance; rationing by selection, as when individuals are accepted for an intervention on the basis of likely benefit or personal influence; rationing by deflection, such as sending people elsewhere to dump the problem in someone else's lap; rationing by deterrence, as when people are put off by unresponsive phone systems, dismissive receptionists, long waiting time, and dismal surroundings; rationing by delay, such as making it difficult to get an appointment; rationing by dilution, by offering less content within any service; and rationing by termination, as when patients are told that nothing more can be done. The authors summarize the idea well when they note that rationing "may be most acceptable when it is not perceived as such: when it represents not so much a consciously taken decision. . . . Lack of supply creates its own lack of demand."[7] Of course, we don't think of the American system as having limitations on supply, but limitations exist, for example in areas with low population density and in specific circumstances, such as hospital nurse staffing limitations to reduce costs, the shortage of nurses and other professionals providing long-term-care services, the absence of psychiatric services in large sections of the country, and the unavailability of child psychiatrists in most places.

If we think in population terms, aggregate health services can be said to be rationed by exclusion of the forty-six million people without insurance from usual care, and the many more who have relatively shallow coverage. However, within our individualized way of thinking, this is not the result of any artificial constraint on supply but simply the result of a lack of capacity to buy. Nonetheless, the problem of uninsurance is one of the prices we pay for a disorganized system in which medical care is better aligned with ability to pay than with need. In the distribution of mental health services and many other types of care, for example, need declines with increased income and education, but service use is directly associated with these indicators of higher socioeconomic status.[8] No other modern nation gives such disproportionate care to those with modest needs while commonly neglecting those who are far sicker.[9]

Rationing Locations

Much of the rationing in modern health systems occurs quietly at two levels. At administrative levels, decisions are made on the content of the program benefits, what will be covered, under what circumstances, and with what limitations.[10] Medicare, Medicaid, and private health plans all make such decisions about what preventive, curative, and rehabilitative elements to include. It is not unusual, for example, for state Medicaid programs to limit mental health and substance abuse services, or to limit the number of prescriptions enrollees can fill in a month. Many private health plans do not pay for many preventive and screening services. Much controversy has involved what some see as lifestyle drugs, discussed earlier, with debates over whether they should be covered, for which patients, and with what limitations on availability. The composition of any benefit design is in part a cultural decision. Some health systems include, for example, rest at a spa as a reasonable health benefit.[11]

Rationing also occurs at the program level and when service is provided. The structure of any health plan establishes the ground rules and the boundaries of what is and is not permissible but leaves much room for discretion for service providers. Among other things, it establishes the benefit design, permissible reimbursable providers and institutions, the resource capacity to respond to demand, and number and locations of providers. It includes such decisions as whether to use drug formularies and whether to have gatekeepers or allow direct access to specialized services. Much discretion devolves to the organized service site, whether that is a hospital, clinic, or other facility.

Managers, living within budgets, have to make decisions on the allocation of personnel; these decisions include the availability of physicians from varying specialties, intensity of nursing services, acceptable waiting times, adoption of new technologies, and the distribution of resources among competing service priorities.

Rationing also occurs at the direct service level as clinicians make decisions about type and intensity of treatment, referral for specialized services, the use of more and less expensive interventions for comparable conditions, and the time and attention to give to each patient. In the American context, what occurs is in part a result of the richness of the patient's insurance, the willingness and ability to pay, and the extent that the clinician serves as an advocate for the needs and wants of the patient. In other systems, for example in the UK, the framework of the health service prescribes no limitation on services, nor does it guarantee particular services. Basically, any service could be available to the extent that resources make its provision possible, and large disparities in the services available in different regions of the UK reflect differential resources and varying local priorities. Since the National Health Service has been chronically underfunded, compared to health services in other European nations, there was a great deal of rationing, but it was implicit for the most part, reflecting the millions of individual decisions made by managers and clinicians in organizing and providing services.

Analysts of the National Health Service talked about an understanding between government and the medical profession to ration care quietly rather than explicitly. Without full awareness among the public of the extent of limitations on what was possible, the health services could function with fewer crises.[12] In recent years this tacit agreement is said to have broken down, and despite vastly increased expenditures on the NHS, the debate about limitations and shortages has become more acrimonious. Also, as patients are better educated and more sophisticated and have access to much more information about what is possible, and care provided elsewhere, patients become more insistent about the availability of specialized services. For example, the earlier policy of the NHS to restrict dialysis for chronic renal failure to younger patients[13] is no longer acceptable. The NHS has little explicit rationing; most rationing occurs by delays in care, waiting lists, and other types of deterrence.

Implicit and Explicit Rationing

An advantage of implicit rationing is that it provides managers and clinicians with discretion to take account of varying life circumstances and preferences. It also reduces public controversies by making exceptions for those who are likely to create public controversies and engage in public confrontations when care they believe should be made available is denied.[14] The darker side is that it tends to give advantages to more educated, sophisticated, demanding, and even obnoxious patients and provides opportunities for the doctor's nonmedical beliefs, prejudices, and discrimination to influence clinical decisions.[15] Such biases have been documented on many occasions. Also, giving clinicians unlimited discretion can introduce large inequalities in allocation of resources. In the NHS, despite obvious resource limitations, GPs could refer patients for any care they thought justified. One London GP referred a patient who made her living as a model for breast enlargement, justifying the decision on the basis of her career needs and the procedure's contribution to her self-esteem. This was generally seen as folly, but justifiable within the operating NHS framework. It is for this reason that many ethicists who have addressed the rationing issue believe that allocation decisions should be open and transparent and involve the public in decision making.[16] Rationing by setting rules beforehand is typically referred to as explicit rationing.

Explicit rationing that forms part of the framework of the health system as in benefit design is more acceptable than explicit rationing applied at the point of service. Individuals in America who acquire different types of health insurance plans may not understand all the particular contingencies, but they are likely to understand that certain types of services like mental health, substance abuse, or long-term-care services may or may not be covered. They are likely to know that spa vacations and elective cosmetic surgery are not part of their plan, but they are less likely to know that particular medications might be excluded from the drug formulary. Explicit rationing, applied at the bedside in the care of individual sick patients, is much more problematic, especially when it clashes with what clinicians believe is in the patient's best interests. This was the case during the 1990s under managed care, when clinicians and patients were explicitly denied specific treatments that clinicians sought for their patients. This type of explicit rationing angered both clinicians and patients, contributed to a strong backlash against HMOs, and resulted in much litigation.[17]

The state of Oregon developed the Oregon Health Plan (OHP), an ambitious effort to establish a framework for explicit rationing to extend its Medicaid program to more enrollees within a restrained budget.[18] The goal was to provide basic and necessary care to a much larger population of eligible persons by distinguishing between more and less useful medical interventions, with the criterion for inclusion defined by what the budget in any year would permit. After a series of public meetings and meetings of advisory groups, medical services were classified into a large number of condition-treatment pairs that were then ranked in terms of judgments of efficacy and other community values, and prioritized. Of the more than 700 categories established, it was initially anticipated that the state budget would allow reimbursement for only 588. The initial formal rankings led to some seemingly absurd outcomes when, for example, tooth capping came out with a higher priority than surgery for ectopic pregnancy or appendectomy, which could be lifesaving.[19] Criticized for violating the "rule of rescue" and for other seeming aberrations, the list was reordered on the basis of clinical experience to correct for the circumstances identified by these criticisms. Although most of those who attended community meetings and participated in the process were health professionals, the process was widely seen as a rational and fair way to make difficult public allocation decisions that rationed less by exclusion of people and more by the value and efficacy of services.

Implemented in 1994, the OHP was able to extend health care to an estimated 320,000 new beneficiaries over the first four years of the plan.[20] But the Oregon rationing process was not what it seemed, or what much of the world commentary seemed to suggest. The extensions in the Medicaid program came mostly from enhanced state funding under improved economic circumstances and by moving heavily into managed care. Since most Medicaid enrollees were receiving care from HMOs and under capitation, providers generally served patients in the manner they believed appropriate and didn't give a great deal of attention to the prioritized list. Moreover, there were many loopholes in the law that allowed physicians who were using the list to provide services below the line to persons who had other treatable conditions above the line.[21] Although observers do not all agree on what actually took place, there is much agreement that little real rationing occurred. The list could be used as an instrument to negotiate capitation rates with HMOs, but ultimately such pricing decisions depended on many factors.

In a provocative analysis Lawrence Jacobs and colleagues argue that the OHP was a political strategy used to bring awareness of medical needs to the legislature and the public and to support enhanced investment in public health services.[22] They note that not only did prioritization not ration service to any appreciable extent, but the process in fact brought about a more generous benefit package than either Medicaid or private insurance had typically offered earlier. Prior to establishment of the OHP, Oregon had one of the most impoverished Medicaid programs in the country, but a growing economy made significant upgrades possible. This allowed policy entrepreneurs to build political momentum, establish community trust, and enlist wide public participation. As they point out, even in the case of transplantation—a dispute that helped initiate the rationing debate when a seven-year-old boy on Medicaid with leukemia was denied a bone marrow transplant—coverage became more generous under the OHP than before, not only in private insurance plans but also in Medicaid.

Tragic Choices

Although much of the cost of medical care is in the moderately expensive things done over and over again millions of times, the rationing debate typically focuses on situations where there is an inability to provide a lifesaving resource to everyone who might benefit, such as in transplantation of hearts, livers, kidneys, and lungs, not only because of cost but also because there are too few organs available. These situations have been termed "tragic choices" because there are disagreements about what is fair in deciding who receives the limited resource and who lives and dies,[23] but there is no "correct" choice. A great variety of criteria have been applied under varying occasions such as allocation by immediate medical need, by age, by the largest opportunity to benefit, by waiting time, by ability to cooperate in treatment, by family circumstances, and even on some occasions by assessments of contributions to the community, but all these criteria raise ethical issues.[24] Even the seemingly medically objective criteria are open to subjective bias, as when judgments about capacity to cooperate in the care process are made on the basis of education, higher intelligence, or attractive personality. An impressive example comes from the area of serious mental illness, where it was widely assumed that persons with schizophrenia and HIV infection would be less capable than others of adhering to the required HIV combination therapy regimen. An empirical study that investigated this question found that people with schizophrenia did not do significantly worse in adherence than people without serious mental illness.[25]

Even within the most well developed and systematic allocation methods, persons of influence find ways to jump the queue as, for example, was alleged but also denied in the case of Mickey Mantle's liver transplant and Governor (of Pennsylvania) Robert Casey's heart and liver transplant. Moreover, with persistence, aggressiveness, and resources and with the help of publicity, some aggressive and demanding patients and families can overturn thoughtful and reasoned decisions.

I was able to observe this process firsthand many years ago when I was teaching at the University of Washington Medical School. I was having lunch with Dr. Belding Scribner, developer of the Scribner shunt, a pioneer in kidney dialysis and chief nephrologist at the medical school. The medical school had recently set up the first chronic dialysis unit for patients with end-stage renal disease, but access to the dialysis unit was very limited. The unit had developed a committee evaluation process with community representatives to allocate these lifesaving but scarce places. Our lunch was interrupted by one of the associate deans, who indicated that Senator Warren Magnuson had been on the phone asking that a friend have access to one of the scarce places. This powerful senator had been a friend of the university and had helped bring much funding to the medical school, but it was unclear that access for his friend could be achieved through the established process. While we sat there, a plan was launched to bypass the usual allocation process by making this patient a special research subject. Many years have passed, and we are now more conscious of the ethics of these endeavors, but it is still true that the rich and powerful, if sufficiently motivated, may find their way in. It should be noted that the initial allocation process established to make these difficult decisions in Washington became a source of embarrassment when it became known that decisions were being made based on such criteria as whether a patient attended church.

A highly publicized case in England illustrates another aspect of the issue, where the services are not unavailable but the cost to the public purse relative to the expected benefit appears excessive. This case involving a ten-year-old child with myeloid leukemia who had previously received two courses of chemotherapy and a bone marrow transplant occasioned much discussion.[26] She suffered a relapse in 1995 and was expected to die in six to eight weeks without treatment, which would have cost about $120,000 at the time. The physicians in charge of her care saw little hope and believed that further treatment was not in her interest. The health authority refused to fund the additional requested "last chance treatment," leading the father to sue. There was considerable confusion about the possibility of the child improving with further treatment; physicians' estimates varied from as little as 1 to 2 percent to as high as 10 to 20 percent from some physicians the father contacted in the United States and elsewhere. An initial court decision asserted that where "the question is whether the life of a 10-year old child might be saved, by however slim a chance, the responsible authority must . . . do more than toll the bell of tight resources."[27] The decision was overturned on appeal; the higher court deemed it inappropriate for judges to second-guess medical services on the difficult and agonizing judgments that had to be made "as to how a limited budget could be best allocated for the maximum advantage of the maximum number of patients." A private donor made it possible for the treatment to go forward, but the child died.

This particular case received more attention than many others, but it is characteristic of numerous cases where patients sued health plans after being denied an allegedly lifesaving procedure, as in litigation over denials of bone marrow transplants for women with breast cancer. Although courts sometimes required plans to provide the service, or unfavorable publicity led plans to retreat from their initial decisions, subsequent studies showed the transplants to have no value for the condition.[28]

The fact of the matter is that despite the call by many ethicists for rationing to be explicit and transparent, this is in fact extremely difficult to carry out, since it mobilizes disease advocates and professional interest groups and results in considerable political conflict. It should be no surprise that the Oregon Health Plan discussion began with the denial of a bone marrow transplant and that the explicit refusal to provide a further bone marrow transplant to a ten-year-old child in England led to a protracted discussion in the press and in policy journals. In reality, there is little explicit rationing at the service level, with the exception of services that many see as marginal to basic health care, such as cosmetic procedures, tattoo removal, in vitro fertilization, and payment for what some view as enhancement drugs like Viagra.[29] Even these limitations, when they are explicit, have led to significant debate over whether denial of the service can have serious social and health costs. Thus, in the case of exclusion of tattoo removal, critics have pointed to visible tattoos shared among gang members in prison that mark the person as a deviant and are said to seriously harm community reentry and life chances following incarceration. In short, the argument is that any limitations should be implicit depending on the doctor's clinical judgment and on a dialogue between doctor and patient.

Setting Limits Fairly

Whatever the realities of medical possibilities and cost constraints, there is little consensus on criteria for allocation of care or for the legitimacy of rationing itself. Some are not alarmed about the growing proportion of GNP going to health care because they see it as a worthwhile expenditure. Most are supportive of ridding the system of waste and worthless interventions, but it is impossible to cut waste without at the same time sometimes restricting worthwhile services. Even more basic to future allocation discussions is the fact that in many instances the distinction is not simply between a worthless expenditure and a worthwhile one. It is a decision about value for money, and people especially disagree when there is some good in the additional service although the cost for what is received may be exorbitant. Clearly, we need a framework for making such decisions meaningfully and in a manner that has public acceptability. We lack such a framework, but work by Norman Daniels and James Sabin is contributing toward a methodology that makes progress on this score.[30]

Daniels and Sabin have been working with HMOs and health plans to establish an approach to setting limits fairly, with the understanding that the imposition of any limits involves both winners and losers. Thus, for such limit setting to work, people must trust the system and accept the legitimacy of the processes through which determinations are made. The core concept to these analysts is what they call "accountability for reasonableness," and such accountability is seen as having four elements. First, they maintain, decisions and their underlying rationales must be public and easily accessible. Second, these decisions must be based on evidence, principles, and justifications that all participants can agree are relevant to decisions about how to meet diverse needs with restrained resources. The evidence need not prove the case in definitive ways, since there is often some uncertainty, but it should reasonably support the decisions made. Third, limit-setting decisions should be open to challenge, should be revisable in light of further information, arguments, and experience, and there should be clear mechanisms for appealing and revising decisions. Finally, there must be a regulatory process in place that can monitor how the process proceeds and ensure that the conditions of information accessibility, relevance of rationales, and processes for revision are all in place.

The framework has been useful to national governments with centralized health care programs as they decide on allocation priorities. Its implementation in the American context is more difficult, with many competing interests at stake, professionals who have a history of clinical autonomy that they strongly value, patients who want what they want when they want it, and organizations themselves functioning under public gaze and in situations of greater market competition, much government regulation, and a high prevalence of litigation. Most organizations don't seek to gain the distinction of rationing elegantly or even to be noticed as rationing at all. Nevertheless, the Daniels/Sabin paradigm can work quite well for what can be seen as smaller rationing decisions. For example, Daniels[31] offers the example of prescriptions for SSRIs for the treatment of depression; there are many choices, but none demonstrated to be any more effective for the average patient than Fluoxetine (Prozac), which is now available generically. Basing its decision on a controlled study and physician prescribing habits demonstrating no special advantage for any SSRI, the Kaiser Permanente pharmacy policy board introduced a generic fluoxetine-first policy. A fail-safe in the Kaiser Permanente system is that physicians retain the authority without prior review to override any restriction they feel is not in their patients' interest. However, variations in prescribing patterns are not large, and a peer culture has developed respecting policy decisions of this type.

We see useful progress in some of the large health plans and in some large medical groups, but, as with many emerging innovations, diffusion and creating culture change are difficult and slow processes. There remains much cultural resistance to making many of the difficult choices that need making. The public seems willing to accept more readily many of the distortions in insurance coverage, gaps in access to care, social disparities, and iatrogenic conditions that result in part from the continued belief that establishing limits is unnecessary and an affront to our individual rights. There are those who tell us that the real issue isn't costs and expenditures but improving decision making and quality, and that solutions depend on one or another innovation such as giving patients more responsibility, providing more information about how hospitals and clinicians perform, paying for performance, or computerizing medical records. Given the momentum in medical knowledge and technology and medical entrepreneurialism, it is inevitable that we will be required to make difficult choices. We need to do all we can to prepare ourselves to make them in reasonable ways that can achieve public legitimacy.

We pay an extraordinarily high price for our reluctance to allocate care more thoughtfully and fairly. The inequities in access and provision of high-quality care contribute to our embarrassingly poor performance on morbidity and mortality indicators compared with countries that are much less affluent. People lose not only by having too little care but also by receiving too much unneeded care, with the risk of injuries resulting from health care itself. Demand on government for more unrestricted health care provision and the rapid growth of health care expenditures compete with other important priorities and make it less likely that those priorities will be adequately financed. The need to pay more for health care requires employers to limit wages and makes it difficult for individuals and families to balance their budgets. And despite the trade-offs between wages and salaries, total compensation packages, particularly in companies with aging workforces and many retirees receiving health benefits, make companies less competitive in global markets and more motivated to outsource work. Beyond the failure to get value for money, the willingness of our society to tolerate the health disenfranchisement of much of the population and the maldistribution of services in relation to need undermine a sense of community and furthers divisions between socioeconomic groups, races, age groups, and geographic areas.

Chapter 9

Restoring Trust in the Health System

Opinion polling is often limited in a way that leaves much to the imagination and to the respondents' interpretations. But in a national survey in 2002, the National Opinion Research Corporation posed a detailed question to respondents about their willingness to accept their physician's judgment.[1] The survey asked:

> Imagine you've been experiencing headaches. You visit your doctor and talk to him about your symptoms. You also tell the doctor that you've been feeling a lot of stress lately. After doing a complete examination, the doctor decided that the headaches are probably due to stress. You want to have an MRI to make sure everything is okay. An MRI is a special and expensive type of x-ray that allows doctors to take detailed pictures of parts of the body such as the heart, spinal cord, or head. Remember that after your complete examination that doctor thinks you don't need the MRI. Then imagine you have the following conversation with the doctor about the MRI and financial incentives.

In this dialogue, the patient speaks first.

> Patient: I'd feel better if I had an MRI. I'm worried that you won't order it because it is too expensive.
> Doctor: I can understand that you're worried whether everything is OK. It also sounds like you're worried that I'm not ordering the test because it's too expensive. These days with managed care lots of people share your worries about this. I want to set your mind at rest because I truly do not think the test is needed at this point . . .

Respondents are then asked: How much would you trust the doctor to put your health above costs? Would you say . . . completely, mostly, somewhat, a little, or not at all?

The responses to this question are distributed broadly, with only two-fifths completely or mostly trusting the doctor and almost one-fifth not trusting the doctor at all. As noted in previous chapters, perhaps the most significant challenge in future medical care is to align growing technological opportunities and new medical interventions with the resources reasonably available to provide care. This is likely to be the case in the future particularly in programs like Medicare and Medicaid, which are financed substantially by tax revenues. The problem is not simply the extent to which very expensive and untested interventions are used and the enormous waste encouraged by financing incentives. Increasingly, concern also focuses on expenditures that provide small, marginal benefits at much increased cost.

Our medical care arrangements and the cultural and economic activities that shape them pose uncertainties and dilemmas for even casual patients, no less for those whose lives and welfare depend on their care. Should one purchase health insurance, and which plan will best fit one's needs? Should one opt for some of the new plan products, such as medical savings accounts or other consumer driven health options? When should one begin thinking about long-term-care insurance, and is such insurance a good purchase? How can one meaningfully compare and judge the plans available? Where should one get

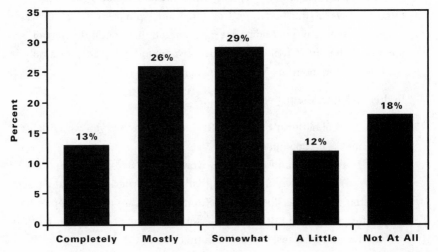

NORC Survey Results on Trusting Doctor

health care? When facing serious illness, how much confidence should one place in one's primary caretakers? How can one reconcile what one is told when it conflicts with information from the media, the Internet, or direct-to-consumer advertising? Should one simply go to the hospital one's doctor recommends or should one attempt to identify a hospital that provides the highest quality of care? Can one put much faith in the ratings and other information available? Should one do what one's doctors suggest or seek further guidance, and from whom? And so on. Ultimately, the question comes down to whom one can trust in making health care choices and decisions. There is much evidence that trust in the traditional authorities the public depended on in the past has eroded significantly. Trust, however, is key to an effective health care system.

Why Is Trust Important?

Life would be quite impossible if we couldn't trust that most people we deal with on a daily basis behave as we expect consistent with their roles, responsibilities, and relationships to us. Similarly, life would be very difficult if the less personal organizations and institutions we must deal with commonly failed to meet our expectations. We all understand that deviance and betrayal occasionally occur in personal relationships, and organizational malfeasance is not rare, but we hope and anticipate that these patterns are disruptions from normal states and not the usual state of affairs. In most activities—whether driving in traffic, banking, purchasing stocks, filling prescriptions, or using public transportation—where we have transactions with people we don't personally know, in order to get along reasonably we must assume that the norms and regulations in place to ensure order and responsible behavior will protect us from exploitation and harm. We know it is quite possible that another driver might disregard red lights and potentially threaten our lives, but we can't reasonably stop at every intersection to make sure that doesn't happen. We have to trust that the rules of the road are in place.

Trust involves expectations of how individuals and institutions will behave in their transactions with us, and it always involves risk, because there is no certainty. In many interactions the stakes are trivial and we can trust easily and not be much harmed if we are wrong. But the stakes also can be high and involve our fortunes, reputations, self-esteem, and even our lives. Being treated badly, and even lied to by an occasional storekeeper, may be no big deal; being lied to or betrayed by a lover, spouse, or dear friend is. Putting up with an incompetent and unresponsive telephone company, airline office, or automobile dealership may be frustrating and even a bit costly, but depending when one is seriously ill on an incompetent and unresponsive doctor or dysfunctional hospital involves bigger stakes.

Medical care is an aggregation of both small- and big-stake transactions, but trust is particularly important in patient-doctor relationships because of the intimate nature of aspects of taking medical history, physical examinations, and treatment; the effectiveness of the relationship may depend on the patient revealing intimate and privileged information. Also, successful treatment often depends on patients' cooperation and willingness to adhere to medical advice. Patients who distrust are less likely to share important information or follow the doctor's advice. Distrustful patients are also less likely to attain value such as encouragement, emotional support, and realistic optimism from the relationship. Misplaced trust can be costly, but to get the advantages of trust one has to assume some of the risks.

Trust is typically strongest in what sociologists call primary relationships, those built on sustained interaction over time among persons who are part of an interconnected constellation of relationships. Trust in that context is not only built on a continuing history of relationships and expected future interactions but also the knowledge that failure to meet one's obligations will have implications for the entire web of associations. Thus, most people believe they can trust family and kin more than acquaintances and strangers. As communities have become more complex and individuals more mobile, we inevitably are increasingly involved in secondary relationships and have a greater need to put our trust in strangers and impersonal organizations and institutions. The historical transitions of moving from small and more intimate communities to larger, more impersonal associations, and the consequences of these transitions, have been at the core of sociological inquiry for generations.

Medical care involves important primary and secondary relationships. People must depend on the competence and integrity of large impersonal structures like health plans, health sciences centers. and hospitals. But most also aspire to have a more personal relationship with their regular physicians, one in which doctor and patient develop a history together, feel secure in their expectations, and have a sense of loyalty to one another. When there is trust between patient and doctor, communication proceeds more smoothly and usually more effectively. It is hoped that the doctor will become the patient's guide in dealing with secondary medical institutions and relationships and help facilitate the relationships between the patient and medical strangers.

Trust is an issue of concern in medical care because people have much less trust in medical leaders and the medical system than they once did. This is not necessarily a bad thing, since some of the earlier trust was misplaced and medical leaders often were more concerned with their own interests than that of their public. Excessive cynicism and distrust, however, interfere with effectiveness and make it more difficult to correct many of the problems our health system faces now and in the future. The fragmentation of medicine itself and competition among specialties, institutions, and medical organizations make it difficult to identify anyone who speaks authoritatively for medicine.

Factors Associated with Loss of Trust

The problem of trust in medicine is part of a much larger issue of trust in social institutions and related to globalization, the growth of the media and its influence, and societal changes around the world.[2] No social institution has been immune from attack or, at times, from erosion of public confidence, and the pattern seen in the United States is common around the world. Depending on time, place, and the immediate circumstances, any social institution may be higher or lower in public trust.

Medicine in the United States in its golden age, from the end of World War II to about 1970, held a special place in public respect and admiration, only surpassed by such august institutions as the U.S. Supreme Court.[3] Over much of the twentieth century medicine had, through a variety of astute measures as described in Paul Starr's Pulitzer Prize–winning volume, *The Social Transformation of American Medicine*,[4] established dominance over medical care and other health care professions. Medical leaders attained quasi-official powers in regulating the practice of medicine, presented a united voice, and often punished physicians who deviated from the party line, such as those who accepted employment in HMOs. Attaining good standing in the medical community required membership in the local medical society, and in those earlier days this required a linked membership in the American Medical Association. People respected doctors and medical achievements and heard few dissenting voices or criticisms of doctors. Doctors were loath to testify in malpractice suits, and lawyers were unwilling to sue doctors. As late as the mid-1960s, three-quarters of the American population expressed confidence in medical leaders, compared with only about half who expressed trust in leaders of other major social institutions.[5]

In the mid-1960s confidence in the federal government and most other institutions began to fall precipitously for many reasons; perhaps the most important was the war in Vietnam. It was in this period that public distrust of experts mounted and willingness to express dissent over government policy grew impressively. In the 1950s and early 1960s, approximately three-quarters of those surveyed said they trusted government, but by the mid-1970s it was approximately one-third.[6] Among the attitudes associated with loss in confidence was the belief that government was run by big interests looking out for themselves, that public officials don't care what people like me think, and that quite a few people running government are crooked.[7]

Most other institutions suffered a similar fate in loss of public confidence; by 2002, only about a one-third of the public had confidence in major institutions such as government, business, labor, and the press. Confidence in medical leaders suffered a similar fate, falling sharply between 1966 and 1976 and continuing to fall, although more slowly, since then.[8] Medicine retained some advantage over other institutions, since it had a larger distance to fall, but by the late 1990s medical leaders shared low standing with leaders of other major institutions. Social trust has much eroded in modern society, but personal trust in agents of at least some institutions has eroded much less. While most people have a low opinion of the American Congress, most people trust their specific member of Congress.[9] Similarly, while people hold many negative beliefs about medical leaders and medicine as an institution, most trust their personal physicians. During the approximate period when trust in medical leaders was falling, surveys found little loss in patient faith in their doctors or in their satisfaction with care.[10] Studies of patients noted increased questioning of doctors and some erosion of confidence in the doctor's authority, but the more significant pattern was the large gap between what people thought about medical leaders and doctors in the abstract and what they said about their own doctor and experiences.

Types of Trust and Their Determinants

In recent years much has been written about trust, and many analytic distinctions have been suggested. For our purposes, three will be adequate in exploring trust in physicians and medical care: trust as a disposition, interpersonal trust, and social trust.

Trust as a Disposition

We recognize that some people are more trustful than others, more willing to accept what others say and do, and less believing that others are out to cheat or deceive them. Some of these differences may be temperamental, others influenced by early upbringing, life experiences, or cultural beliefs. We tend to view such personal inclinations as part of the person, more as psychological attributes than social ones, but even this disposition is very much influenced by the social context. Surveys have asked respondents for many years the same question of whether they believe most people can be trusted. This belief generally is seen as an indicator of personal disposition. Ironically, responses can vary a great deal from year to year; for example, in 1960, 58 percent of those surveyed said most people can be trusted, but only 37 percent agreed in 1993.[11] We know that some people we deal with seem paranoid, but even paranoia can be influenced and shaped by current events, media suggestion and reinforcements, and shared beliefs. Doctors worry about seemingly paranoid patients. They may disclose less useful information and are less inclined to cooperate in treatment; doctors also fear that such patients may be more inclined to sue them. In some environments, physicians worry about their personal safety.

Interpersonal Trust

Interpersonal trust relates to the individual expectations people have about their relational partners. It derives from the trust people first develop with intimates and kin, which then extends to other relationships. It is the stuff that social scientists write about under many labels, from *gemeinshaft* to primary group relations to, more recently, social capital.[12] Trust in one's doctor, particularly when one is seriously ill, has many of the attributes found in trusting relationships within primary groups.

When patients report on their trust in various aspects of medical care, their most salient concern is how much they trust their physician. In beginning a new relationship with a doctor, they bring their past experiences, with varying beliefs and dispositions. Most people in America believe that sufficient controls exist in medical training and in licensing to ensure that most doctors are reasonably competent, and many enter new physician relationships with initial trust in the doctor.[13] But patients in studies also tell us that while they trust, they also seek to ensure that their assumptions are correct. Some go even further, devising simple tests to assess doctor reactions and determine whether initial trust is well placed.[14] Trust is further enhanced when the doctor has been recommended by another trusted doctor or health professional, when the doctor has a good reputation in the community and particularly among family, friends, and acquaintances, and when the patient has chosen the doctor rather than having the doctor assigned in some way.[15] Trust is an iterative resource that grows over time as patients have more opportunities to assess how doctors respond with changing circumstances. Patients typically develop more trust with continuity of care.

People who have serious illness often face situations and uncertainties that lead them to be more dissatisfied with their medical care and with their physicians. Serious illness makes the patient more dependent on the doctor, which puts the patient at greater risk should the doctor not respond appropriately. Serious illness can lead to building very strong trust or, alternatively, to disappointment in how the doctor responds and an erosion of trust. Patients vary in response when their trust is violated: they may do nothing; they may complain, they may change doctors, or they may take a combination of actions. A good doctor-patient relationship is much valued by patients, and many patients are unwilling to complain, or cautious in their complaints, because they want to protect the doctor's loyalty for future occasions when they feel they will need it.

Patient trust is generally focused on three aspects of care: the doctor's technical competence, the doctor's interpersonal competence, and the doctor's commitment to the patient's welfare.[16] There are other dimensions, especially important to some patients, such as confidentiality and disclosure of conflict of interest,[17] but these are much less salient. It isn't that patients don't care about confidentiality, but most assume that doctors will treat information about them and their disease as privileged information.[18] They are aware that information may leak through clerical staff or in other ways, but we have yet to encounter a patient who assesses trust in their doctor by the efforts the doctor makes to train and supervise staff on such issues as confidentiality.

There is, of course, a large inequality between patients and their doctors on technical issues, but patients often have beliefs based on their experiences and what they learn from the media, friends, and the Internet. Many patients also believe that in some sense they are experts on their own body. As a start, they see technical competence in the reputation of the doctor, the doctor's training and qualifications and other credentials, and the doctor's intellect. Many judge expertise and intellect by indications that the doctor keeps current, thinks ahead, has new information, and double-checks to ensure accuracy. But for the most part, as I will explain, much of the subsequent assessment of technical expertise is derived from interpersonal cues. Patients also judge doctors, often erroneously, by the fact that they weren't getting better, seemed to be getting worse, that the medication prescribed didn't work and may have had adverse effects. Patients also not infrequently criticize doctors for having misdiagnosed them. At a deeper level, patient narratives reveal that many have difficulty coping with the uncertainties of medical care and some may blame doctors inappropriately. In contrast, some research suggests that patients are generally accurate in their assessments about the quality of care they are receiving.[19]

The interpersonal competence of physicians is central in evaluating and trusting them. Patients properly put a great deal of emphasis on interpersonal behaviors that they can make reasonable judgments about. Core to interpersonal competence is evidence of listening, caring, being concerned, and showing compassion. When one analyzes the behaviors that lead patients to these judgments it is striking that these are not intangible personality qualities (what has been commonly called "the art of medicine"), but mostly teachable skills.[20] Obviously some doctors are temperamentally warmer and more empathic than others, but much of what goes on is modifiable with proper training. Patients describe doctors who lack these critical interpersonal skills as condescending, abrupt, patronizing, arrogant, and distracted. In contrast, those perceived as having interpersonal skills are seen as more friendly, respectful, truthful, responsible, attentive, reassuring, sensitive, and nonjudgmental. One common skill patients comment about is whether doctors make eye contact.

Above all, patients want their doctors to be their agents and to be committed to their welfare. Patients are not unrealistic and understand that doctors face constraints, but they want their doctors on their side, willing to advocate and fight for them when needed. This is not simply a response to managed care, although it is relevant to it. Many patients interviewed in our studies do not really understand in any developed way the various organizational and financial pressures on their doctors or the types of conflicts that some doctors may face under some managed care relationships. The notion of the doctor fighting on their side, and in their interests, transcends these newer developments in medical care. In fact, when some of the financial conflicts that doctors face under some capitation arrangements are explained to patients, many vigorously disapprove. Patients do not want to see their doctor as just one more service worker or businessman. They especially value what they see as the special professionalism that defines the physician.[21]

Social Trust

Social trust refers to trust in larger organizational entities, such as group practices, health plans, hospitals, and health care systems. Such trust may relate to personal experiences one has had or be secondhand through the experiences of family, friends, and acquaintances. It may be based on incidental contact with some small segment of a larger organization or on more sustained experience with it. Social trust may also be based on no personal experience at all but formed through the media, advertisements, and reputational scuttlebutt. Most people can tell you that the Mayo Clinic is a fine institution, but they can't tell you much about why it is.

The quality of health care depends very much on how care is organized, how health facilities select, train, supervise, and monitor their employees and professionals, and the quality-assurance systems in place. In many instances having the right organizational arrangements is as important or more than having the right doctor.[22] Patients and doctors continue to think largely in terms of personal relationships rather than in terms of the organization of care. Patients commonly believe that if they have the right doctor, this doctor will guide them through the larger system of care, get them to the right specialists and hospitals, and generally ensure that their interests are looked after. They assume that when their doctors choose a specialty referral, they are selecting an appropriately competent person and that they can transfer their trust, at least initially, to the extended relationship. The assumption that their doctor has the knowledge and influence to predict and control the subsequent trajectory of care is commonly wrong, as many patients with serious illness come to understand. The patient's health plan, physician practice structure, hospital, nursing home, and home care agency can make a great difference in what transpires.

Health plans, hospitals, and specialized facilities compete for patients in part by advertising the quality of their doctors and specialized capacities. They gain prestige by having on their staff doctors who are known to be outstanding, or who at least gain recognition by their research reputations or organizational or media ratings. Similarly, doctors gain credibility by their associations with esteemed institutions.[23] One may know little about a specific doctor, but the fact that he or she is affiliated with the Mayo Clinic or the Johns Hopkins Medical School may give patients the confidence to trust. The assumption is that such institutions seek to select only the best doctors and demand high quality of care from them. This is not a completely erroneous view, but knowing the size, complexity, heterogeneity, and decentralization of such institutions should make clear that reputation may not alone provide the desired protection or justify the confidence that patients seek.

Disrupted Trust

In larger and more complex societies people must have transactions with many people with whom they have no personal history and for whom they have no strong basis for trust. Moreover, the stakes involved in these transactions can be significant, as employees and others who lost most of their pensions or savings discovered. In commerce, we generally understand the principle of let the buyer beware, but how do we protect ourselves from immoral bankers, stock brokers, lawyers, developers, food producers, builders, real estate agents, and many more in a position to take advantage of us? When personal trust is lacking or diminished and the stakes are high, legal and regulatory agencies must develop mechanisms that are substitutes for trust, that allow people to be confident that they can enter transactions with less risk, and that facilitate social and commercial transactions.[24] Thus, for example, the federal government guarantees bank accounts so people will trust their banks enough to deposit money in their bank accounts rather than keeping their money under their mattresses. These regulations are further buttressed by professional norms and ethics that seek to assure the public that practitioners maintain a high standard and that peers will police one another and punish transgressors.

Medical care has many mechanisms that help build trust and restore it when it is damaged. These mechanisms involve the body of medical ethics taught to aspiring doctors, the various tests and procedures required for licensing and certification, the many laws and regulations pertaining to medical negligence, hospital safety, the proper dispensing of medicines, and so on. When new issues arise, legislatures commonly respond with new rules and procedures, as they did with the growth of managed care. As public dissatisfaction with managed care mounted, many states passed legislation requiring grievance procedures, independent reviews of disputes, minimal hospital stays for childbirth and mastectomy, and a variety of other patient protections. Congress debated a Patient's Bill of Rights for several years but never successfully passed one, but such rights were extended by several state legislatures. Following the thalidomide tragedy in which an anti-nausea drug taken by pregnant women in many countries, although not in the United States, led to the birth of many deformed babies, procedures for evaluating the safety and effectiveness of drugs by the Food and Drug Administration was significantly strengthened. With increasing concern over the marketing and excessive use of potentially harmful drugs like Vioxx, this may soon happen again. Concerns about the misuse of patient information led to new elaborate privacy protections. Concerns about the proper use of human subjects led to an elaborate system of institutional review boards and procedures to assess risks and benefits for research volunteers and the adequacy of informed consent procedures. Physician conflicts of interest also are defined by legislation.[25]

Some look back to the time when a handshake was better than a contract, and when people felt they could trust partners in a transaction to meet their obligations. But as transactions become increasingly segmented and impersonal, most important transactions are managed more formally. Contracts are a means of giving partners assurance they each understand their obligations. Contracts, of course, can be litigated when disputes arise, but litigation is expensive, time consuming, and often stressful. Lawyers who have studied how contracts function have noted that they are often not enforced legally but serve as a basis of informal negotiation when differences occur.[26]

Thus, contracts serve as much to promote trust as templates for legal action. The parties know that they can always go to court when all else fails.

Regulations, appropriately applied, can be very helpful in giving participants the assurance that matters will proceed as expected. The downside of these regulations is that medicine is extraordinarily complicated and it is often difficult to write good general rules. Thus, legislators and regulators develop new rules for each emerging problem, developing an elaborate web of regulations that become burdensome and costly for all involved. Each new rule may seem to make sense in dealing with a specific problem, but the totality often creates conflicts and contradictions that were unanticipated when the rules were first developed. It was not the intent of malpractice regulations to encourage doctors to do procedures they thought of no use other than to protect themselves against litigation, leading them to practice what we call defensive medicine. It was not the intent of staffing regulations in mental institutions to encourage these institutions to discharge patients prematurely and inappropriately, abandoning them in order to meet the required staff-patient ratios. It was not the intent of research ethics committees to make consent requirements so demanding that they discouraged research subjects from participating in research that involved little risk, or encouraged researchers to avoid some difficult topics entirely. And so on. Regulation is necessary for many reasons, but it is important to remember that rules have costs as well as benefits and their cost-effectiveness needs scrutiny.

Explaining the Loss of Public Trust

The erosion of trust in social institutions is a generic problem that has become increasingly common around the world. While trust fluctuates from one country and period to another, and among institutional sectors, its course in contemporary societies is generally downward. Erosion of trust is a manifestation of global societies, instant access to information, multiple and conflicting informational sources, continuing disputes about and disconfirmation of core values, and competing and conflicting interests that are more apparent than ever before.[27] The media compete aggressively for markets, and the public seems less drawn to positive reports than to those detailing disasters, mayhem, conflict, dishonesty, and violations of trust. For example, while people say they dislike negative political ads, these ads seem to work for many candidates. It takes great effort to build social trust, but one extraordinary abuse or scandal can quickly destroy it. Modern media dwell on the negative, leaving the public with the sense that the world is a troublesome place and dangers await us at every turn.

We live in an age of celebrities but not of heroes. Respect for expertise was diminished by the Vietnam War when some of the "best and the brightest" lied to us continuously; they continue to do so.[28] Even medical scientists, who were typically seen as disinterested in their search for truth and desire to help humanity, are now so compromised by financial interests that their integrity is increasingly called in question.[29] Universities and scientists, seen perhaps as among the last bastions of honest inquiry, have become hungry for money, and some compromise their core values.[30] The pharmaceutical industry, once seen as more ethical than other industries, engages in research manipulation and marketing practices that many view as dishonest and that are sometimes unlawful. It is no surprise that pharmaceutical companies now rival tobacco companies and HMOs in lack of public respect.

The erosion of trust in part reflects the reality of an increasingly competitive marketplace, of which medicine and health are major components. One can debate traditionalists' claims that privatization and profit have destroyed the virtues of medicine,[31] but there is little disagreement about marketing hyperbole and the jockeying of health plans, hospitals, and specialist groups to capture market share and enhance their remuneration and profits, or about the many efforts made to game the reimbursement system and to market selectively to attract low-risk patients. Medicine can no longer speak with a united voice because specialties increasingly compete among themselves to gain control over particular medical turf, and to gain advantageous reimbursement from government and health plans.[32] And, typically, they go where the money is, as has been evident in the growth of specialized cardiovascular and orthopedic hospitals. These are areas where reimbursement has been generous, but the separation of these more lucrative areas drains community general hospitals of the profits that allow them to subsidize under-reimbursed services or care for the poor and the uninsured.[33] Congress and state legislatures are awash with health lobbyists promoting the interests of groups of every type, and as in defense, energy, and many other areas of social policy, health policy makers move readily between government and special interest organizations.

On the other side, the public is better educated than ever before, and rightfully more skeptical of authoritative claims. The public has extraordinary access to information. While many do not exploit informational opportunities and are not well informed, it is difficult, given the character of the media, to fail to understand that medicine and the health system face many difficulties, that medical experts have varied opinions on most matters that patients care about, and that poor care, waste, fraud, and abuse are not uncommon. While a great deal of good goes on in our medical care system, the overall picture drawn by the media is quite negative. Most people remain satisfied with their personal physicians and the care they receive, leaving a large gap between their own experience and their general perception.

Building Trust in Medicine and Medical Institutions

Many medical leaders and medical professional organizations are alarmed by the erosion of social trust, and even by the much smaller loss of authority on the part of people's personal physicians. Most patients are still rather docile, but these days more patients talk back. They demand particular treatments they have learned about and do not accept their physician as final authority. Those who are more educated increasingly demand to be partners in their own care, insist that they be informed about treatment options and participate in decision making, and increasingly come to medical care armed with treatment information from the Internet and other media. Patient advocacy groups are of great importance and have fundamentally influenced how care and even research are undertaken, for example, as in the treatment of AIDS and breast cancer.[34] Medical leaders understand that times have changed and that if they are to recapture the trust they once had they will have to find new ways of relating to patients and the public. A variety of initiatives are in place or being planned, including a range of professional and ethical educational activities sponsored by a number of major medical organizations.

Large organized group practices have done better than small local practices in adapting to change, and some have demonstrated the innovative possibilities of systems to identify problems early, prevent errors, manage chronic diseases more effectively, and provide educational opportunities for patients. Such organizations as Health Partners in Minnesota, Kaiser Permanente on the West Coast, the Group Health Cooperative of Puget Sound in Seattle, and the medical system administered by the VA have demonstrated the value of many of these ways of caring for patients.[35] In an effort to better understand what was happening, particularly as it pertained to trust, Marsha Rosenthal and I surveyed medical directors from all HMOs in the United States in 1996.[36] HMOs start with some disadvantages on the trust issue, because they tend to limit a patent's choice of physicians and hospitals. These restrictions on choice are one of the features of the prepaid group practice HMOs patients most dislike. Even these traditional HMOs now commonly offer point-of-service options that cover care outside established networks, but at greater financial cost to the patient. Most medical directors who responded to our survey saw trust as a major concern. More than two-thirds indicated that trust was a prominent factor in designing their administrative strategies, and more than three-fifths indicated that they emphasized issues of trust in communicating with professionals and other personnel in their organizations.

More specifically, we asked about a range of organizational programs related to trust that we had learned about in earlier interviews with HMO administrators and professionals. Almost all the HMOs had specific efforts to improve patient satisfaction, and patient surveys and focus groups were very commonly used. A majority saw these efforts as very useful. Other common arrangements that were seen as particularly beneficial included using mediation for dispute resolution, formal support programs for patients and their families, and patient representatives and ombudsperson programs. We found that group/staff HMO models were most likely to have this kind of program to build trust, an observation consistent with the existing literature. Two factors might be particularly relevant in explaining this. First, such group/staff models have tighter management and can more readily introduce such programs. Second, because group/staff models tend to be more restrictive of patient choice, they may feel a greater need to have such programs. We also found, consistent with the work of others, that nonprofit HMOs and those not affiliated with a chain were more supportive of public service and community programs, the types of programs that transcend direct provision of care to enrollees.[37]

Various national medical organizations are increasingly concerned with issues of trust and medical professionalism and have been searching for ways to address these concerns. In 2002 the Foundation of the American Board of Internal Medicine, the American College of Physicians, and the European Federation of Internal Medicine disseminated a Charter on Medical Professionalism endorsed by a large number of medical organizations in the United States and around the world.[38] The charter addresses the principles of social justice and patient welfare and autonomy. It defines ten professional responsibilities including commitment to professional competence, maintaining appropriate relationships with patients, improving access and the quality of care, and seeking a just distribution of resources. Making the charter more than a statement of aspirations, however, requires concrete translations of these responsibilities in specific contexts and road maps that help physicians understand how these obligations can be exercised in the face of everyday realities. Disseminating ethical aspirations and giving them greater visibility is a start. The profession's sincere interest in promoting these principles, and efforts to implement them more specifically in certification and recertification requirements, also may modestly contribute to public confidence to the extent the public is made aware of these efforts.

Medical specialties have in more recent years moved to address some of the evident problems of safety and medical error, and there are signs of increased subspecialty cooperation. All the American Board of Medical Specialty boards have moved toward a lifetime learning perspective and are setting up requirements for physicians to maintain continuing certification. Initiatives include standardizing credentialing and cross-specialty training and evaluation to improve quality of care. As Rosemary Stevens, a renowned scholar and participant in these efforts, has noted, "ABMS-approved specialty boards are trying to improve standards for communication with patients and peers, professionalism, and effectiveness under the maintenance-of-certification program, which all boards have endorsed."[39]

Taken singly, none of the measures is likely to have much impact compared to the powerful influences that are challenging social trust in medicine. But in combination, efforts to increase access to care, the use of electronic medical records, new quality-assurance programs, efforts to reduce medical and hospital error, more sophisticated management of chronic disease, holding medical students, residents, and practicing physicians accountable for conflicts of interest and ethical lapses, and building a renewed culture of medical professionalism have great value. Only the future can tell how much we succeed in transforming the current culture of medicine and medical work.

The Fork in the Road

Public views of the U.S. health care system have been monitored since 1986, and surveyors report that at any given time one-half to three-fifths of the population believes the system has good points but that major changes are needed to make it work better.[1] In 2003 only 11 to 13 percent reported that the system worked pretty well and that only minor changes were needed. In the same year, 30 percent believed the system needed to be completely rebuilt. In a national survey in August 2005, respondents ranked health care as the second most important problem that government needed to address, behind only the Iraq war and foreign policy.[2] The vast majority of the population agrees that major changes are warranted. This is less than the historic high in the early 1990s prior to the debate over the Clinton health care plan, but these data over some years reflect a public willingness to consider change. The problem is that those who have acceptable insurance and care are loath to forego what they have. If they come to believe that changes would diminish their personal situation, they choose the status quo. Also, many draw back at any suggestion that changes would increase their personal tax burden to any appreciable degree. Groups opposed to health care changes quite readily play on these fears and have had success in mobilizing opposition. Although the Harry and Louise TV ads during the debate on the Clinton reforms may have not been as important as some believe, they reflect the strategy of playing on people's fears and on their distrust in government. From 1992 through 1994 only one-fifth of persons polled trusted the government in Washington to do what was right always or most of the time.[3]

Despite people's seeming receptivity to change in the medical system, experience has shown that it is difficult to mobilize the population in a united way and relatively easy to fragment their support. Many powerful advocacy organizations become involved, each protecting its interests and constituencies, leaving no politically persuasive active majority. It is probably true that if conditions are perceived as bad enough and the efforts for reform are led by persuasive and credible leaders and effective coalitions, significant change could occur, but neither the current context nor the credibility of leadership suggests that we are anywhere near the threshold.

Although there is no indication of major breakthroughs in the next several years, there is much concern about the issues examined in this book, and broad desire to take steps toward improved performance and outcomes. We may bemoan the inability to arrive politically at an overall solution, but there are many steps we can take to close insurance gaps, increase access to care, reduce disparities, improve quality, enhance population health, limit medical error, ensure the safety of drugs, and much more. We have to make sure that our more global aspirations do not become the enemy of the good. Review of the past history of health reform politics illustrates how unwillingness to compromise among competing forces resulted in stalemate and significant lost opportunities. In the two chapters that follow I explore some of the many ways we might move forward, whatever our political ideologies and personal preferences. The pressing task at this particular time is to muddle through as elegantly and consistently as we can.

Chapter 10

The Challenge of Change

There is widespread agreement that major changes are needed in our health care system but little consensus on how to achieve them. Strong philosophical differences about the appropriate responsibilities of the public and private sectors, how care should be financed, the roles of consumers, providers, payers, government, interest organizations, and other issues discussed throughout this book divide policy makers, interested participants, and the general public. While some may await the next political opportunity to make the case for a major overhaul of the health care system and a program of national health insurance, neither our health policy history nor political and economic trends make this a promising likelihood in the foreseeable future. The failures to resolve comprehensive reform efforts when economic and political conditions were more favorable suggests that we might do better to think incrementally and in a way that invites greater collaboration across the ideological divide. It may be a lot easier to get agreement on enhancements of coverage, quality, and safety issues, for example, than on broad philosophical concepts of health care rights and responsibilities.

There is in fact much that Americans agree on despite their political and philosophical differences. There is broad consensus that good health and health care are prerequisites for fair life chances and that everyone should have access to appropriate medical resources. Such views are particularly strong in the case of more dependent populations such as children, the elderly, and persons with disabilities. Moreover, most believe that the availability of medical care should be based on need and not simply social status or the ability to pay. Most people also believe that disparities in access to health care based on race, ethnicity, or other social distinctions are inherently unfair. Although there are different views on how much care should be publicly subsidized, most agree that no one should be denied basic services or be forced into bankruptcy by bills for catastrophic care. There is also broad consensus that fraud and waste should be reduced, that medical error should be eliminated to the extent possible, that care should be responsive and of high quality, and that it should be easier to navigate the health care system.

Covering the Uninsured

The overarching challenge is how to ensure that all Americans have at least basic health coverage.[1] There has been no shortage of proposals, including national health insurance provided through a federal program like Medicare; requiring employers to provide coverage or taxing them if they do not ("pay or play"); mandating that individuals purchase insurance and subsidizing such purchases among persons with low incomes; providing tax credits to individuals and employers for insurance coverage; covering more people by means of expanding government programs such as Medicare (for retired persons under age sixty-five), Medicaid, the State Children's Health Insurance Program (SCHIP); and many approaches that blend several of these ideas.

Complicating the debate about mechanisms are the historical American skepticism toward large government programs, concerns about how employer mandates affect business profitability and jobs, resistance to individual mandates that are seen as encroaching on individual freedoms, and concern about increased tax burdens from expanding government programs. Yet we are already paying many of these costs through creative cost shifting, since we provide much free care to people in need and prohibit hospitals from turning people away in emergencies regardless of their ability to pay. By delaying care until people suffer major illness episodes and treating health problems in an episodic way through emergency rooms and fragmented outpatient departments in clinics and hospitals, we promote inefficiencies and the excessive use of high-cost providers. Failure to provide more comprehensive care results in much unnecessary illness and death. The current financing system is basically unfair, since employers who provide health insurance for their employees and those people who buy private insurance in the individual market partly subsidize the care of employees whose employers do not provide insurance. Similarly, hospitals that provide a great deal of free care subsidize those that provide little or none. Although federal disproportionate share payments and state charity programs compensate some institutions that provide indigent care, these payments only cover part of the costs.

Underlying the insurance debate are strong beliefs about deserving and less deserving populations, viewpoints that go back to the early English Poor Laws that sought to enforce strong individual responsibility. These orientations persist in concerns about people who are "free riders" and beliefs that individuals should be responsible for contributing their share and not simply depend on public provision. Linking the level of subsidy to family income helps deal with such concerns. One way to proceed that would garner considerable bipartisan support would be to work vigorously to enroll uninsured children who are eligible for public programs like Medicaid and the State Children's Health Insurance Program (SCHIP). Some states have done much better than others. We have to take the approaches developed and lessons learned from successful states and implement them more widely. As of 2003, more than eight million children had no health insurance coverage, and one-third of these children received no medical care during the year. Some 70 percent of uninsured children who are eligible for these programs still are not enrolled.[2] Additional children can be covered by expanding Medicaid and SCHIP for children to higher-income thresholds. A 2000/2001 study of children under eighteen years of age found that 6.6 percent had no insurance and an additional 7.7 percent had insurance for only part of the year.[3] Children with no insurance and with gaps in coverage were more likely to have unmet needs, to have care delayed, to have fewer preventive visits, and to have unfilled prescriptions.

Low-income parents can also be incorporated into these programs as state financing permits. A significant problem for states has been the large increase in Medicaid costs. Given the way insurance is structured, concern remains that extending public benefits to expanded populations would provide incentives for employers and workers to drop private coverage and shift responsibility to the public sector. Extending care to more children is a relatively low cost component of public programs; disproportionate expenditures go for long-term care for the poor elderly and disabled populations, which are smaller. Children make up about half of eligible enrollees but consume only about one-fifth of the cost. This leads many who support universal insurance to advocate starting with children, because they are attractive recipients from a public standpoint, and not very costly to insure. Since many uninsured children are in families with a working parent, providing incentives to employers to cover uninsured families can help in the interim.[4] A Wal-Mart memo made public in 2005 revealed that 46 percent of the children of Wal-Mart employees were uninsured or on Medicaid. Some children will remain uninsured under any of these scenarios, and continuing support and expansion of the community health center network and other children's programs such as school health and public health clinics and outreach can help provide preventive and other basic services.

Another major gap in insurance involves early retirees who do not have coverage through former employers. Many retirees find it difficult to purchase insurance at reasonable cost in the private individual insurance marketplace. Allowing retirees to buy into the Medicare program offers a more efficient way for this group to gain coverage. One of the largest uninsured groups is young people who are in the process of embarking on a work career and are not yet settled but who lose their parental coverage because of age limitations. This subgroup tends to be quite healthy, and most are not in need of much expensive medical care. Since the cost of purchasing insurance in the private individual market can be exorbitant, many do not purchase coverage. Developing more ways to facilitate extended coverage under parental insurance, creating specialized insurance-purchasing pools for this population, and providing low- or no-interest loans for purchase of health insurance would help get more of these transitional young adults insured. There are other critical subgroups, such as the unemployed, who also require special targeted approaches.

All of these expansions would require state and federal revenues and must contend with public and political resistance to increased taxes. This has been a major barrier to more comprehensive proposals but also pertains to each of the types of expansions discussed. Incremental change that takes place outside large political and ideological debates is easier to enact and offers more realistic opportunities in the near term. The process is untidy and difficult and inevitably results in gaps, but it allows progress to be made in steps as more comprehensive but more contentious proposals gestate in the background. The reality is that given the political divisions in the country, proposals for change have to be indeterminate to some degree, leaving room for important interest groups to believe that they and their constituents have something to gain or, at least, will not be big losers.

Promotion of Evidence-Based Practices

Almost everyone supports the idea of evidence-based practice in the abstract, but its implementation has been slower than this consensus suggests. Part of the problem is the complexity and uncertainty of much of medical knowledge; contending interests have a stake in integrating the evidence differently. Doctors and patients hold to their views that appropriate decisions about care for any individual patient should be made in the context of the unique circumstances that define that patient's needs. Moreover, many practice recommendations are based on judgments of cost-effectiveness, but in any given instance doctor and patient may prefer treatment that is believed to be advantageous even if it is excessively expensive relative to alternatives. Many interventions are not totally worthless but offer little value relative to their costs, and patients and doctors may insist on the intervention nevertheless. There is sufficient knowledge in many areas of medical practice to help doctors and patients arrive at a thoughtful course of treatment less influenced by hype and advertising, but time pressures and the complexity of the informational environment make it difficult to draw reliably on this large knowledge base.

Significant government incentives will be necessary to overcome economic and psychological barriers to adopting new information technologies, but such expenditures would help build the practice infrastructures needed to make evidence-based medicine more a reality, put in place better disease-management programs, and implement other ideas such as pay-for-performance. Developing a national health information network, however, is a very expensive venture that will require large investments from public and private sources. One expert panel has estimated that such a system would require a capital investment of $156 billion over five years, and $48 billion for annual operations.[5] While the federal government has made some modest financial investments toward a health IT network, the creation of such a network is unlikely to occur without much larger federal participation.

Important to the evidence-based effort is building credible ways to evaluate the quality of research, study biases, and applicability of research to patients different from those studied in randomized controlled trials and other studies. Such credible evaluators can offer the best informed consensus on the state of current knowledge. Many public and private organizations are attempting to do this, but it is necessary for them to collaborate on a strategy and speak with fewer but more credible voices. An independent organization with impeccable scientific credentials, and with public participation, could play a central role, perhaps using the UK's NICE as a model. The organization might be structured along the lines of the Federal Reserve, working closely with government but more insulated from everyday politics than typical government agencies. We already know from past experience that several government agencies designed to do this were not sufficiently protected in carrying out this difficult function.[6] To the extent that a credible process can be developed, we can anticipate that large insurers would join government in efforts to implement the best scientific advice about treatment efficacy. Other possibilities might include a role for organizations like the Institute of Medicine of the National Academies of Science, which can mobilize the needed expertise and bring to the table representatives of government, private insurers, health care organizations, and medical professionals. Although at this point we are far from having a recognized mechanism for making these difficult decisions, insulated from ideological, political, and economic influences, private organizations like Consumers Union (CU) have high credibility with the public. While CU is selectively addressing some medical issues such as the drug cost information noted earlier, the tasks are much larger and more complex than an organization of this type can realistically deal with.

Many methodological questions remain in amassing and reviewing the results from the world literature. Randomized controlled trials (RCTs), while the gold standard, can vary a great deal in quality of design, size, and appropriateness of sample; attrition and other biases; the range of process and outcome measures evaluated; the length of time patients are followed; the fidelity of the intervention; and much more. Randomization protects against selection biases, but studies based on nonrandomized methodologies, if carefully designed and carried out, can also be helpful. This is particularly the case in evaluating multifaceted interventions on social care and psychosocial services, which have to be tailored to some degree to particular patient needs, preferences, and circumstances. There are also important cautions relating to the validity of subgroup analyses within RCTs, where the effects were not initially predicted, and misleading inferences can result from data mining in the search for significant correlations. Many such associations and chance findings that were not predicted and have no plausible biological basis are commonly communicated to the public by the media and encourage wasteful and even dangerous health practices. As publicized risks change from one week to another, the public understandably becomes skeptical of the underlying science. This contributes to inattention and neglect of good scientific results that could make a real difference in people's lives. Publication bias also remains a serious problem, because not all trial results are reported and those that are may misrepresent the overall picture. Meta-analysis of RCTs, a methodology to bring together the findings from all studies on a particular issue, attempts to capture unpublished data, but this effort typically is uncertain and incomplete. The uncertainties in analyzing the state of evidence make it crucial that evaluators be unbiased, have no conflicts of interest, and have high credibility.

There are serious practical problems in assessing medical and surgical interventions that make them more difficult to assess than drugs. Research is a slow process, and results often become available after new interventions have been changed or perfected. While approval of drugs and medical devices must await initial research findings on safety and efficacy, this is not true of new treatments, including new surgical interventions. When studies find uncertain or no benefits, innovators or their commercial sponsors commonly argue that the intervention has evolved and improved and the research findings no longer apply to current practice. It seems reasonable, however, that the burden of proof should lie with those who make claims for new and expensive treatments. Health programs should not pay for interventions not yet demonstrated to have value except in the context of RCTs and other research studies. The history of bone marrow transplants in the treatment of breast cancer and many other medical and surgical interventions that when appropriately studied were found to have no value should encourage caution. Doctors and patients demanded this very expensive therapy, sometimes going to the courts to reverse coverage denials by health plans. Yet when appropriately evaluated, bone marrow transplant was found to be ineffective and probably substantially diminished the quality of life of patients who received this procedure.[7]

Evidence-based practice is an evolving movement. It depends on the education of new cohorts of physicians and other health professionals, and the perspectives they will bring to their work. As new cohorts complete medical school and residency training, they increasingly will have assimilated an evidence-based perspective and will feel more comfortable with the new technologies that make implementation more possible. Compared with those physicians in a transition time who see the conditions of practice changing under their feet, later cohorts will take many of these new arrangements for granted, especially if medical school and graduate medical education appropriately perform their roles.

Reinvigorating Primary Care and the Chronic Care Challenge

One of the deficiencies of American health care is the continuing erosion of the primary care role and the loss of the kind of continuing overall health management and continuity that builds on the knowledge of individual patients and their needs. Relatively low reimbursement exacerbates the growing frustrations associated with the increasing expectations of primary care clinicians and growing administrative complexities. It is no surprise that young physicians, attuned to a different lifestyle than earlier cohorts, are increasingly attracted to specialty practice. Rebuilding primary care will require attention to the structures of practice that allow doctors to care for patients in more interesting and effective ways, that relieve them of some of the unnecessary burdens that are common in practice, and that compensate them more fairly relative to specialty practice.

We have no assurance that aspiring doctors in the future will select primary care over specialty practice. As more women make up the future physician workforce both here and abroad, they also will prefer work conditions that limit their hours of continuing responsibilities, and some medical roles are more demanding than others. National health systems such as England's NHS can shape occupational distribution by controlling the proportion of specialist practices and closing overdoctored areas to new primary care practices. Also, concerned that many woman doctors would not choose primary care because of the schedules that interfere with family life, the NHS has made it more possible for GPs to opt out of after-hours care. Maintaining this kind of direct control over specialty positions, practice location, and practice conditions is not acceptable in the United States. Instead, we can seek to make primary care more attractive through improved reimbursement and organizational changes that make such roles more professionally fulfilling. The introduction of new information technologies and disease-management systems, the extension of care through teamwork and use of nurse practitioners, physician assistants, clinical pharmacists and other personnel, and the development of a continuing learning environment as part of the practice culture can all help make primary care seem less like a treadmill and more professionally rewarding.

Large organized group practices, particularly prepaid groups, are in many ways the most favorable context for introducing these practice improvements and developing new evidence-based innovations. However, such organizations are uncommon in most of the United States, and most doctors, even those in HMOs, still function in small groups, which may have contracts with a number of large health plans. It is considerably more difficult for small groups to take advantage of new technologies and teams, or to invest the resources in disease and practice management systems that are being developed in large, innovative organized settings. However, many private vendors are organizing programs focused on chronic disease-management with nurse management services that can help on many of these tasks; with time these systems will increase in accessibility and quality.[8] The technologies are developing rapidly and will eventually make it possible to undertake impressive monitoring and patient educational initiatives. Our concepts of how to provide excellent primary care and chronic disease management will continue to evolve, but primary care must remain a vital part of health care delivery in the United States. One possibility is to have available a variety of primary care alternatives, including the nurse practitioner as the clinician of first contact and continuing care.

The Chronic Care Model

Innovators of chronic care models, in contrast to the prevalent acute care ori-entation, have been advocating changes in how we provide care for decades. But they have had only isolated success because of deficiencies in the provider systems, clinical information technology, and opportunities to provide support for physician and patient decision making. Many of the innovations, as already noted, occurred in the large prepaid groups or large systems that provided more multidisciplinary care and practice infrastructure than was typical in the mainstream system. One of the innovative leaders in chronic care was the Group Health Cooperative (GHC) of Puget Sound, the source of a number of demonstrations and research evaluations of disease management and the chronic disease model. Dr. Edward Wagner, who was associated with GHC and involved in these programs, went on with the support of The Robert Wood Johnson Foundation to direct a Foundation program to disseminate the model in physician group practices and community health centers.[9] This model has a number of elements, among them the use of teams to improve care of patients with chronic illness, case management of the sickest patients, education and support for patients and families in understanding their illnesses, self-care (including the use of patient support groups), and increased use of emerging technologies for sharing information and help in getting information to make informed decisions. Such information technology assists teams as they moni-tor patient progress and helps guide practice in an effective, evidence-based fashion. Such tools also make it more possible to include patients as serious participants in their own care.

It is difficult to know the extent of diffusion of this chronic care model, although Wagner has reported that five hundred physician groups have imple-mented at least some of its components.[10] The chronic disease model repre-sents a perspective on care more than a formula and will vary by the type of disease and disability, and the tools available to any particular provider group. As we have already noted, few groups have the full information and decision support technology available, or have as yet the scale to organize the kinds of multidisciplinary teams found in larger organizations and health centers. Proper management of chronic disease requires that each group have a registry of persons with each of the major chronic diseases so they know who they are, can monitor their progress, can provide appropriate reminders and prompts, and can intervene in a timely way when needed. Now that Congress has directed the Centers for Medicare and Medicaid Services to address the issue as part of the Medicare Prescription Drug Improvement and Modernization Act of 2003, and insurers and other organizations have taken greater interest, there is growing momentum for this perspective. But as noted throughout this book, incentives have to be appropriately aligned, organizations have to work together, and the organizational and technological infrastructures have to be put in place.

As Lawrence Casalino has observed, there are two dominant pathways to achieve appropriate management of chronic disease: either through the clinical group itself or by enlisting the participation of a disease-management company to work with patients in a complementary way. These organizations monitor the patient's progress, help with self-monitoring and care, provide patient education and social support, and communicate to patients' doctors when specific medical interventions are needed.[11] Although the disease-management industry is small, it has been growing. Disease-management companies mine data from administrative data sets and clinical information and can build systems and programs for larger populations than most physician groups serve. The downside of this approach is that it segments the management process from the care process, setting up potential competition with doctors, coordination problems, and potential lack of cooperation. One of the basic ideas of the chronic disease perspective is to overcome fragmentation and integrate multidisciplinary services. It remains to be seen how effectively disease-management companies can work with individual physician groups to realize the potential of a chronic disease perspective.

Many of the problems reviewed throughout this discussion are linked to each other in important ways. The segmentation of care and lack of coordination, for example, are related to poor chronic care management, reduced quality of care, and the occurrence of medical error. A recent study in Minnesota of drug errors in seventy-eight medical group practices found that 28 percent of the prescriptions written and reviewed by the researchers involved some kind of error. Many of these errors involved overdoses. Using more restrictive criteria (prescriptions involving adverse drug interactions, having two similar drugs prescribed for the same illness, abuse of controlled substances, and contraindicated prescriptions because the patient had other chronic diseases), 13 percent of filled prescriptions were in error. The researchers also found that group practices that used case managers had lower error rates. and they concluded "that poor coordination of care from multiple providers is one of the root causes of drug errors."[12]

The Pharmaceutical Challenge

There has been much contentious debate about pharmaceutical issues and policies, made more visible by the new Medicare prescription coverage, the high cost of drugs, the interest among states and many consumers in purchasing drugs from abroad, where they are considerably less expensive, and the need to withdraw major drugs from the market because of unanticipated serious side effects and negative outcomes. Much has been written on the calcium-channel blockers as a first-choice treatment for hypertension, Vioxx and other Cox-2 inhibitors for arthritis, phen-fen for losing weight, the potential dangers of SSRIs in treating depression in children, and much more to alert the public that serious dangers lurk behind the promotion, marketing, and prescription of drugs. A great many important pharmaceutical issues have been and will continue to be actively debated for years to come and are highly contentious. They encompass such issues as incentives for drug development, patent policies, safety and efficacy regulation, the promotion and marketing of drugs (including direct-to-consumer advertising), post-marketing regulation, the cost of drugs, and drug formularies. Here I focus briefly on just a few of these important issues.[13]

The debate will continue as to whether drug regulation in the past inappropriately delayed the approval of new drugs, thus harming patients who could have benefited, or whether the focus has tilted too far toward approving potentially dangerous and harmful drugs before their safety and efficacy are properly assessed. Nor is there much consensus about using industry fees to fund a significant part of the FDA budget for evaluating drugs. Some critics believe that this makes the FDA too dependent on industry and more likely to defer to it. The data remain unclear about the balance of costs and benefits of quicker or slower drug approval processes, but it is clear that initial FDA reviews cannot adequately assess less frequent dangers until the drug is used by larger numbers of people, and for longer time periods than would be included in clinical trials prior to approval. Thus, post-marketing studies are essential; they should be required as part of the drug-approval process and should be enforced, monitored, and regulated. The editors of the *Journal of the American Medical Association* have urged a major restructuring of the post-marketing surveillance system, including the decoupling of the drug-approval process from post-marketing monitoring and regulation. They believe manufacturers "should be required to conduct clinical studies to assure safety for all products" and that "protocols for adequately powered post marketing studies be mandated at the time a new drug is launched."[14] The Vioxx example is one of the more recent publicized cases of the importance of post-marketing surveillance, but it is also indicative of broader policy issues that need to be addressed.[15] With greater vigilance and transparency of research results, the harmful effects of Cox-2 inhibitors, and particularly

Vioxx, would have been widely known by 2000, several years before the issue was widely appreciated.

The public has not understood that the FDA evaluates the efficacy of a new drug relative to a placebo, and not in relation to already marketed medications. Thus, drugs can be approved that are not only no better than existing drugs but are inferior to them. The pharmaceutical companies have become big marketing enterprises that can take new drugs of little added value and by aggressively marketing them to physicians, hospitals, and consumers can achieve enormous sales. For decades, critics have documented the nefarious promotional practices of pharmaceutical companies, which provide meals, entertainment, and even vacations under the guise of education for doctors, who learn much of what they know about new drugs from biased marketing promotions. It is unlikely in the American context that we are going to interfere with marketing practices that are not illegal or grossly deceptive, so other approaches will be needed, such as unbiased public detailing and more accessible public information. However, we should consider whether it is appropriate to raise the standard for new drug approvals to at least a level of requiring them to be as efficacious and safe as existing medications. Patients may react differently to drugs in the same class, so such regulation would have to be flexible and take into account the need for alternatives.

Some will argue that any such change would be anticompetitive, establishing monopolies for already existing drugs and inhibiting innovation. Drug purchasing, however, departs substantially from a competitive marketplace, and "me-too" patented drugs are typically marketed at prices many times greater than their generic equivalents. Demand for these brands is stimulated by aggressive promotion practices. The physician is, in theory, the prudent purchaser for the patient, who cannot acquire the drug without a prescription, but most physicians are not sufficiently informed about either the price or other comparative advantages of various drug alternatives. In addition, many physicians acquiesce to patient demands for specific drugs because they do not want to alienate patients or take the time to change patients' views.

Cost of drugs is perhaps the most contentious drug issue, and here again it is difficult to resolve conflicting claims. The pharmaceutical industry defends its prices on the basis of the research and development costs of new drugs, while critics see these costs as exaggerated, and the much higher profits of the pharmaceutical industry compared with other industries as unjustified and achieved in part by political donations and effective lobbying. (Pharmaceutical industry profits are typically about three times the 5 percent median of all industries.) The critics note that most new, innovative drugs are now developed by small biotech companies, which then license large drug companies to produce and market their discoveries. Moreover, critics argue, most of the basic research that leads to drug innovation is funded by the NIH and tax revenue. They emphasize that most new medications in recent years have been "me-too" drugs of little added value, and the pharmaceutical industry has put its primary energies and enormous financial resources less into innovation and more into marketing. Whatever the contending opinions, U.S. patients pay more for their drugs than patients elsewhere in the world, and U.S. consumers provide most pharmaceutical profits.

Whether or not drug prices realistically reflect the research and development costs necessary for innovation, the United States subsidizes the rest of the world by the high prices it pays. Most industrialized countries establish the prices they will pay, or use their bargaining leverage to purchase drugs more cheaply, as do large HMOs, the VA, and state Medicaid programs. When Congress, in enacting a Medicare prescription plan, prohibited the Medicare program from using its purchasing power to bargain down drug costs, it introduced a very large subsidy to the pharmaceutical industry. Medicare is a powerful purchasing entity and should exercise its purchasing power thoughtfully, but this prohibition is counterproductive and should be reversed. Ironically, Congress already uses government purchasing power, via Medicare, to control hospital and medical prices, so it is difficult to see why the highly profitable pharmaceutical industry should be exempt. It is proper for the United States to subsidize medications in poor and developing countries on a thoughtful and targeted basis, but it should not necessarily subsidize other rich nations that pay much less for pharmaceuticals than we do.

The high cost of drugs is not solely an issue for government. Many other participants need to play a responsible role. Although direct-to-consumer advertising receives a great deal of attention, the vast majority of marketing is done to doctors, many of whom rationalize their acceptance of favors.[16] Many have taken significant gifts, and some have profited in corrupt ways, but most simply have accepted modest gratuities, deluding themselves that these trips, dinners, and gifts do not bias their prescribing practices. Physicians both as individuals and through their professional organizations must stop accepting these inducements and condemn the obvious conflicts of interest that tarnish medical professionalism and public confidence.

Increasingly, medical leaders are speaking out on these issues, and medical organizations are beginning to develop ethical standards for what is and is not legitimate, but they too are compromised. The American College of Physicians (ACP), which views itself as a highly professional organization, refused to allow the nonprofit health professional group No Free Lunch, which advocates reducing medical conflicts of interest, to rent a booth at its annual meeting. The ACP reportedly said that No Free Lunch would inhibit dialogue between industry exhibitors and doctors.[17] If this is the response of the ACP, one can only imagine the barriers to overcoming pharmaceutical industry money. The ACP was eventually shamed into reversing its decision. Similarly, residency and continuing medical education programs have come to depend too much on drug company handouts and need to find alternate ways of funding their activities. Physicians have to participate in supporting drug information approaches that are more objective than those currently in use. Patients also have to learn to be more prudent, to understand that there is not a pill to heal every ache, and to be more skeptical about the advertising claims they hear. They also have to be more open to advice from their doctors that the drugs they demand are not necessarily in their best interest. Tiered pharmaceutical benefits that require patients to pay more for expensive brand-name alternatives may help encourage more thoughtful decision making.

Tackling Administrative Costs

People who experience any significant illness are often amazed at the amount of paper this generates. This is particularly the case for those who retain traditional types of health insurance where separate bills and statements may come from health insurer, primary care doctor, each specialty service, the hospital, laboratories, medical device suppliers, and the like. Depending on the deductible and co-insurance, transactions may involve separate interactions with the insurer and a range of providers, and the flow of bills may go on for months. This particular component of administrative costs, only the tip of the iceberg that the patient can see, is a small part of the enormous costs for the system as a whole, reflecting its pluralism, complexity, choice options, reimbursement arrangements, and competition among insurers and providers. While some believe that estimates of administrative costs exceeding 30 percent are exaggerated, few would contend that the vast amounts spent on administrative costs provide value for money.

A major component of administrative cost is the price we must pay for having the type of medical care system we have. By providing a wide range of choice, by providing health insurance in many different forms and contexts, by using co-insurance and deductibles, and by developing very complex ways of paying doctors and other providers, we compound our administrative costs. It is estimated that in 1999 we spent almost twice as much as Canada's national health insurance system (31 percent of health care expenditures, compared with 16.7 percent).[18] Centralized systems are much more easily administered. Medicare administrative costs are only 2 to 3 percent of expenditures, although the Medicare program benefits from administrative expenditures elsewhere in the system. Similarly, large HMOs have comparatively low administrative costs, on average below 10 percent; Kaiser Permanente, the prepaid group program serving eight million enrollees, has administrative costs much lower than the HMO average. The worst offender on the administrative side is the individual insurance market, with its extensive individual marketing, medical underwriting, and insurance agent commissions, which can eat up almost half of the medical care dollar. Woolhandler and colleagues estimate that U.S. administrative health costs per person in 1999 were $1,059. They further estimate that between 1969 and 1999, administrative workers grew from 18 to 27 percent of U.S. health workers.[19]

Administrative costs come in many forms and can overlap with functions related to quality assessment, tracking of the health system, and improving the quality of care. Thorpe[20] has distinguished four major functions embedded in administrative costs: those that are transaction related such as claims processing and billing; benefits management, including management information systems, plan design, and quality-assurance processes; selling and marketing, including advertising and underwriting; and regulatory compliance involving such matters as required reserves, taxes, and licensing issues. Thus, when we advocate electronic clinical records, improved information systems, disease-management programs, and data to establish clinical performance and effectiveness, we are in part arguing for at least short-term increases in administrative costs. Nevertheless, few seriously doubt that the administrative component of our health care system is inefficient and wasteful.

Reducing administrative costs is difficult because they are generated by millions of different actors, including health plans, professionals, hospitals and other institutions, researchers, and even patients themselves. Obviously, having a universal health insurance program, as most countries have, would significantly reduce many of these costs. The degree of reduction would depend on how standard the benefit package is and the range of options and alternatives offered. Efficiencies can be achieved by consolidating some plans and purchasing groups and by sharing standard methods for a range of functions, from claims processing to quality assurance. Rather than let each small group struggle with issues such as information technology systems, claims processing, evidence-based standards, quality-assurance procedures, and designing incentives, we can make efforts to bring together and coordinate participants who share common objectives and goals and who can benefit from sophisticated technical assistance. It makes little sense for each health plan, institution, and professional group to reinvent the wheel. Those seeking to improve incentives, for example, as in current efforts to develop pay-for-performance-systems, need to work together to develop common standards and approaches. Each group potentially gains when all push in the same direction. This challenge is certainly not easy, but administrative costs remain an area promising significant savings with a more rational and cooperative approach.

Toward Building an Evidence-Based Culture

Changing the health care system in a constructive fashion is no slam-dunk. There is too much at stake and too many competing interests to make change easy. As we learned in the controversy over the Clinton health care proposals, while most participants could understand the need for reforms, few were willing to risk their own individual advantages.[21] This is why change is particularly difficult to accomplish without increasing expenditures, since those who already have advantages dig in deeply to retain them. Typically, major changes are supported by new investment, as is currently the case in efforts to bring general practice in the UK up to modern evidence-based standards and in the subsidies provided to health plans and the pharmaceutical industry by adding prescription drugs to the Medicare program. Historical experience suggests that major institutional change is always associated with increased expenditures, as we learned with the introduction of Medicare and Medicaid.

Achieving some of our aspirations to improve prevention and access to care, to increase quality and responsiveness of services, and to reduce disparities may be possible without massive new financial inputs, because American medical care is already very generously financed and continued growth is anticipated. A core problem is that we have excessive faith in the wonders of new technologies, and other remedies and invest large resources in unproven and often counterproductive therapies.[22] In the absence of good evaluative data, usually as reflected in randomized clinical trials as the appropriate standard, we attribute effectiveness to a myriad of interventions when the credit more properly should be attributed to the body's ability to heal itself and to the fact that clinicians typically see patients at the height of their distress and most would improve whatever the intervention. Also, patient expectations are a powerful force, and the placebo effect often has a large influence on both subjective and physical experience.[23]

American culture has become very focused on health improvement and enhancement, and expectations of medical interventions are extraordinarily optimistic. The population seems more focused on a medical fix than on following the daily diet, exercise, and prudent behavior that could do a great deal to enhance the health of individuals and populations. Medical hype, supported by media interest and attention, reinforces these orientations. Similarly, the financial advantages to many enterprises in promoting their services, products, and interventions reinforce the already high expectations for remedies and cures. Patients have extraordinary confidence in medical technologies, some which are indeed remarkable and lifesaving, and they are willing to assume that the next new thing, whether tested or not, is better for them. This also helps explain the success of alternative medicine. Many influences work in concert to promote much waste and counterproductive care.

It is not clear how one successfully addresses unrealistic expectations. The public cares deeply about the quality of its medical care and believes that quality must be improved. While people may criticize the system or physicians in general, most believe that their physician is their most credible guide to better health. In thinking about their care, patients are more concerned about the possibility that they may be denied a useful intervention than the possibility that a treatment is unnecessary and might do them harm. Physicians who are action oriented also tilt in this direction.

Patients often seek health information from friends and family, the media, and, increasingly, the Internet. Much of the information is distorted and unrealistic, often structured to encourage consumption of untested products and services. More unbiased sources of information will increasingly be available and will be promoted by health plans and government agencies, but these efforts will have to be heard above the crowd. Much must be done to help people learn to search information sources appropriately and to differentiate slick marketing from more objective information.

Increased work is being devoted to developing decision aids that help patients select treatment options for major illnesses and elucidate the risks and benefits of alternatives. Some studies show that when patients are given unbiased presentations of these options, they often select more conservative alternatives than medical hype would encourage.[24] A Cochrane review of eighteen RCTs that met inclusion criteria found that decision aids increased patient knowledge and reduced decisional conflict but did not significantly affect satisfaction. Although such decision aids reduced preferences for major surgery and PSA tests, they did not affect minor surgical or screening test choices.[25] Involving patients in decision making is more complicated than it may first appear, since patients have decidedly different preferences about the extent of their participation. A study of 1,633 breast cancer patients found that patients who felt they had too much participation in the decision process, as well as those who felt they had too little, were less satisfied with their surgery and the decision process. The importance of matching participation to preference is clear from this study.[26] It is essential that clinicians understand that many patients seek their guidance and not simply a neutral stance.

Decision aids are difficult to develop in an unbiased and responsible way, and they are costly to maintain as new knowledge develops. It remains unclear how the production of these instruments can be financed and disseminated when there is no commercial advantage. Health plans and government have a stake in patients making good choices and may ultimately support these efforts appropriately, but the future course is far from clear. These programs inevitably will have to compete with the many forces that have strong incentives to encourage consumption of new drugs, technologies, and interventions.

Changing cultural understanding and trends is always a tricky and uncertain enterprise. People's conceptions and orientations are not easily directed, and many forces compete in efforts to influence them. Thus, while our medical future depends on activated patients who understand the potentials but also the limits of medicine, and health professionals who are motivated to provide care based on the best understanding at the time, this is in no sense inevitable. The challenge is long term and uncharted as new knowledge and technological developments emerge and new economic and political influences come into play.

René Dubos, an eminent microbiologist and environmental activist, was once asked why he called himself a despairing optimist. He replied that he understood the magnitude of the difficulties and that made him despair. But he also knew the extraordinary numbers of people with intelligence and dedication who were working tirelessly to get things right. It was these individuals who made him optimistic about the future.

Chapter 11

Steps in Our Health Future

It has been asserted frequently over the past several decades that significant reform of health care would not come until most Americans were unhappy with their health services and demanded major changes. At the time of Bill Clinton's inauguration as president in 1993, the conditions seemed ripe for such change. Medical costs continued to escalate, more persons were losing their insurance, people felt locked into jobs to retain their health care coverage; Americans felt increasingly insecure about the economy, their jobs, and their health care coverage, and health reform had gained political momentum among the electorate. Although it appeared that we were finally on the threshold, interest groups opposed to the president's proposals were able to sway public opinion to opposition.

Some believe we should be on the threshold again. The uninsured population has increased to some forty-six million, and health care costs have escalated, racing well beyond the economy as a whole. More costs have been transferred to individuals and families by employers and public programs, and people feel increasingly insecure about retaining their insurance and being able to afford needed health care services. For the moment there is not much short-term optimism, but many share the view of Arnold Relman, former editor of the *New England Journal of Medicine*, that "a complete overhaul is inevitable, because in the long run nothing else is likely to work."[1] But we have heard this refrain before and those raking in the advantages don't share the view that health care is in crisis.

For the immediate future, most would have to agree with Republican policy advisor Gail Wilensky's assessment that "there is likely to be little federal (or, for that matter, state) money for major expansions in health care coverage. Democrats and others may challenge extensions of tax reductions and argue that those revenues could easily provide the funds needed to cover the uninsured, but the tax cuts are unlikely to be rolled back."[2] Indeed, with the implementation of the Medicare Modernization Act (MMA) and its large incentives to private health plans and the pharmaceutical industry, we can expect a range of additional efforts to cut back other federal spending for Medicare and Medicaid in coming years. Already, in 2005, $10 billion has been cut from projected Medicaid spending over the next five years, and if the Bush administration had had its way, the cuts would have been larger. This occurs in a context where states are struggling with Medicaid growth and are being forced to cut back on eligibility and coverage.

The Bush administration, through the MMA, continues in its efforts to induce Medicare enrollees into private health plans on the theory—some say illusion—that competition among private plans will eventually help control Medicare expenditures. To induce private plans to enter and stay in the Medicare market, payments to private Medicare Advantage Plans are higher than costs in traditional Medicare, despite the fact that traditional Medicare enrollees are sicker and cost more than those who opt for private plans. Estimates of payments to private plans for 2005 indicate that such payments will be 7.8 percent more for each enrollee in a private plan than a traditional plan— $546 per private-plan enrollee.[3] The excess cost estimate for 2005 was $3.72 billion, approximately the same excess paid to private plans in 2004. Similarly, the prohibition against government bargaining over pharmaceutical prices in Medicare constitutes a massive subsidy to the industry. So, at least in the short run, when the going gets tough, the direction of government subsidies to the private sector makes it even tougher to meet the needs of the most vulnerable Americans.

Much of the recent political debate has been centered on Social Security reform, but the real crisis is managing escalating medical expenditures. Medicare and Medicaid face enormous future cost increases with advances in technology, increasing numbers of enrollees, a morass of overly complex and uncoordinated administrative arrangements, and the lack of effective care management. Medicare, with its forty-two million enrollees, is expected to cost $325 billion in 2005, accounting for 13 percent of the federal budget.[4] As with the health system overall, there is no consensus about rationing care on the basis of what is cost-effective and worth doing. Medicare, despite its many virtues and popularity among the elderly, still basically pays for whatever health professionals choose to do in a traditional way, and it doesn't get adequate value for money. The Medicare program tries to constrain cost through reimbursement approaches such as prospective payment and limits on provider reimbursement, but the political power of hospitals, health professional groups, and their lobbies moderates these constraints. Although the health industry lobbies aggressively and persistently against what it alleges to be inadequate reimbursement that threatens health care, in fact the private managed-care industry typically has been much tougher in bargaining with providers than Medicare has been.

Government strategy, thus, has been to try to induce Medicare enrollees into private plans that are freer to manage care than government is. The subsidies to private plans are intended to encourage these plans to become stable partners in the Medicare market. Private managed-care plans, however, offer few of the constructive care advantages of group prepaid programs like Kaiser-Permanente, and critics believe they are more interested in managing costs than care. Many of the elderly also remain suspicious of private plans because in the past they abandoned many elderly, leaving the program in geographic areas where reimbursement was less advantageous. Although government had ambitious plans for increasing enrollment of the elderly in private plans over the last decade, and such enrollment increased from 8 percent to 16 percent between 1995 and 2000, the abandonment of the elderly by private plans in many markets pushed the trend downward so that by 2003 only 12 percent were enrolled. Only time will tell whether Medicare can eventually convert enrollees from traditional to private care coverage and reach their optimistic projection of 30 percent coverage by 2013, an estimate almost twice as high as the one offered by the Congressional Budget Office.[5] Most of the general population now receives its care from a managed-care plan of some kind, but Medicare remains the last bastion of fee-for-service medicine.

Another frequent proposal to reform Medicare is to convert the program from a guaranteed benefit program to a defined benefit program. Such a program, modeled on the Federal Employees Health Benefits Program, would provide a voucher to enrollees that would cover basic health care coverage but would then offer a menu of options providing different levels of care and amenities. Those who selected more expensive options would have to pay the difference between the basic subsidy and cost of the more expensive option. Under such a system, the traditional plan would be more expensive than most HMO options. Critics see this as a rollback of the Medicare entitlement. They fear that under the pressure of cost increases, the basic benefit would be vulnerable to reductions and would erode over time, resulting in significantly different levels of coverage and care. They see this approach as undermining the universality and equity of Medicare and thus as an approach that would disadvantage lower-income enrollees. Underlying the difficulty of resolving any of these major issues is the lack of trust, which mirrors the prevailing partisan and adversarial politics.

Many other proposals seek to contain costs; these proposals range from raising the age of eligibility for Medicare to taxing the value of the entire Medicare benefit for higher-income recipients, and, at the extreme, to converting Medicare to a means-tested welfare program. Raising the age of eligibility will contribute to the growth of the uninsured and underinsured population as more retirees who have no health retirement benefits from their employers, and especially those with the greatest needs for care because of preexisting conditions, will find it difficult to acquire insurance at a cost they can afford. This proposal will exacerbate the already growing problem of retirees below the age of sixty-five who face difficulty getting health care coverage.

In principle there is little wrong with taxing the value of the Medicare benefit for persons of high income, but this would yield relatively little revenue, and some fear that it might contribute to an erosion of public support for this valued universal entitlement. Converting Medicare to a welfare program, the most extreme option and one not taken very seriously, would not only be greatly unpopular but, more importantly, would push our health system away from universal coverage and thus in the opposite direction from where it should be headed. In all likelihood, Medicare will not be transformed by any single initiative, but rather by muddling through with numerous piecemeal changes adapted from various proposals.

Of course, we already have a health welfare program, Medicaid, which is now the nation's largest and most expensive health program. Covering approximately fifty-three million enrollees, it provides a safety net for the disabled and for many poor children, families, and seniors. As a federal-state partnership, Medicaid operates under a federal framework and a variety of federal mandates, but it can differ radically from one state to another in eligibility, coverage, cost sharing, and reimbursement of providers. Medicaid is not only our national health safety net but also our national long-term-care program for poor seniors and elderly persons who become poor because of long-term-care expenses. At its best, this program provides a more appropriate comprehensive approach to care for people with chronic disease and disability than most private health plans do, and it includes many needed services that private insurance typically does not cover, such as transportation, case management, and rehabilitation services of various kinds. But in many states, Medicaid provides only the minimal safety net, with only the most basic required services, strictly limited eligibility, and tough limits on use. Services that are optional for states include such vital ones as prescription drugs, vision and hearing services, and mental health care. Although only 29 percent of covered persons are optional enrollees, three-fifths of all expenditures are for optional services, most provided to persons with disabilities and the elderly.[6] The fact that the care one can receive depends so substantially on where one lives is the single largest difficulty of the Medicaid program. Federal mandates ensure a basic minimum that some states would not provide on their own, but above this minimum there is much variation. Although the federal government assumes a larger proportion of costs for poor states than for more affluent ones, varying from approximately 75 percent to 50 percent in fiscal year 2006, legislatures in poor states often are unable or unwilling to provide funds to extend optional eligibility and benefits, even though the federal government will assume most of the cost.

The reasons are not hard to understand. Many states have low average incomes, are averse to increased taxes, and, unlike the federal government, are required to balance their budgets each year. Medicaid is a major cost for states as well as for the federal government; it now constitutes more than one-fifth of all state expenditures. It is the single largest component of state budgets, pushing out other important investments such as infrastructure development and higher education. On average, Medicaid now costs states more than K–12 education. States naturally are looking for ways to constrain their Medicaid outlays and to transfer as many costs as possible to the federal government. A battle continues between federal and state bureaucrats over what are legitimate cost-sharing formulas and respective payment obligations. State financial administrators vary in their sophistication and aggressiveness in garnering federal dollars, giving some states advantages over others. State officials also vary in their philosophies about responding to federal mandates and depending on federal monies.

Nevertheless, states require federal assistance for the many services that have been mandated as Medicaid has evolved since 1965. Although Medicare was presumably intended to meet the needs of the elderly population, it actually covers less than half of the elderly's health care needs. There are currently seven million Medicare-Medicaid dual-eligibles among the forty-two million Medicare enrollees. Dual-eligibles, who make up 13 percent of Medicaid enrollees, account for more than two-fifths of all Medicaid spending, including nursing home and other long-term-care expenditures, prescription drugs, and a variety of medical services. In addition, Medicaid is required to cover Medicare premiums, deductibles, and co-insurance for low-income elderly, and health care for persons on Supplemental Security Income (SSI), who are fulfilling the two-year waiting period before gaining eligibility for Medicare. Under the new Medicare prescription plan, dual-eligibles will, as of 2006, receive prescription drug coverage under Part D. States, however, have to return savings to the federal government and fulfill other administrative responsibilities under the new program. Some states maintain that this will cost them more than the amounts saved by transfer of dual-eligibles' drug costs to Medicare.

There have been numerous proposals to restructure Medicaid. Some believe basic restructuring is essential, while others see Medicaid as doing a good job filling the many gaps in our health care system and therefore needing only modest adjustments. From time to time it has been suggested that Medicaid be taken over by the federal government, with states taking responsibility for welfare. More recently, it has been proposed that health services now defined as optional be folded into a block grant to states, with a funding cap on federal payments. But many optional services are central to the more developed state programs, and state officials and advocates fear that caps will result in a reduction of federal responsibility. Optional services are crucial in such areas as mental health, where Medicaid constitutes the most important care system for persons with serious and persistent mental illness, as well as in other types of long-term care. States facing budget problems seek maximum flexibility in administering their programs, but advocates fear that too much state flexibility will erode the floor established by federal requirements.

There is broad understanding that Medicaid is performing an indispensable role, but there is also acknowledgment that some features of the program require modernization. A report[7] prepared for the National Governors Association, suggests a range of areas where change should be considered. These include modifying the federal matching formula to take better account of state fiscal capacity and changing state economic conditions; modernizing the unnecessarily complex eligibility rules linked to the earlier welfare system; adopting benefit rules that would make it easier to extend partial coverage to additional uninsured optional groups; and adjusting some cost-sharing features consistent with expenditure growth. One may or may not agree with any individual suggestion, but it is clear enough that Medicaid could benefit from some adjustments to fit contemporary circumstances better.

Many of the controversies involving Medicaid are about cost, but cost increases are in large part a result of factors external to Medicaid itself.[8] Increases in per capita Medicaid spending in recent years have been considerably below per capita increases in private insurance premiums, and Medicaid has always been a frugal payer compared with Medicare and private health insurance. Its parsimony has been a problem in that many providers refuse to participate in the program because of low reimbursement. The cost increases in Medicaid are largely due to substantially increased caseloads resulting from economic factors that have increased poverty, need, and the number of un-insured people in American society. The overall poverty rate increased to 12.7 percent in 2004, the fifth consecutive year of increases in poverty. Also, demand for Medicaid long-term care continues to grow in the absence of alternative policy solutions. The poor elderly and persons with disabilities who require long-term care, although constituting a minority of enrollees, account for much of the expenditure. Medicaid remains an essential program and fills in many places where our health system fails. Given the problems it takes on, Medicaid could do with more rather than less investment. At its core, the real issue involves values and how meeting the needs of the vulnerable shapes up against tax cuts and other government outlays.

In June 2005 the National Governors Association issued a bipartisan preliminary policy reform report that builds on earlier recommendations.[9] It urged that states have the flexibility to shape programs in terms of their particular needs, including providing different insurance products to different populations, allowing greater co-insurance and deductibles, allowing states more authority to negotiate prescription drug costs, and making it easier for the states to receive waivers and make changes in the program. Indeed, the report urges a federal statute eliminating the waiver process needed to make many changes. The report addresses a range of reforms from large and contentious ones, such as relieving Medicaid of financing the long-term-care costs of dual Medicare/Medicaid eligibles and having Medicare or Social Security take on long-term-care funding, to less contentious ones, such as making it more difficult for elders to transfer financial assets to gain eligibility for Medicaid long-term-care services. Beyond these more specific issues, the report argues for broader restructuring of health care, including more incentives for personal responsibility, more flexible insurance programs for the nondisabled population so that the programs would more closely resemble the model of the State Children's Health Insurance Program than traditional Medicaid, and efforts to strengthen employer-based and private health care coverage. Governors are clearly alarmed about their growing Medicaid costs, but this is only the first stage of many discussions over several years about how to hold Medicaid in check.

The future of our health system requires timely replenishment of health facilities, work force, and technology. Each generation of new doctors, nurses, and other health professionals must be trained and socialized in the light of new knowledge and developments. There have been growing concerns about future physician supply, but the problem is likely to be more about willingness to perform generalist roles and locate in rural areas than about supply per se. Practicing medicine, whatever the complaints, remains a highly attractive profession that is both economically and personally rewarding. While older doctors who have seen the conditions of their work change rapidly gripe a lot, doctors now entering medicine take many of these changed work conditions for granted. Persons entering medicine today also have different perspectives and orientations than in earlier times and feel differently about working in group settings, time commitments, schedules, and levels of responsibility. The large increase in women in medicine also involves changes in views about preferred work settings and specialty selection. Women also practice differently than men, giving more attention to communication and patient relationships.

The quality of patient care depends greatly on nursing, and the future of nursing remains a significant challenge. The fastest-growing area in nursing has been in the training of nurse practitioners and nurse specialists who have enhanced expertise and take on added responsibility. Nurse practitioners are assuming more primary care responsibilities and providing more chronic disease care, often in independent and quasi-independent roles, and this is likely to accelerate in coming years. Nurse practitioners and physician assistants can prescribe medications in a number of states, and they increasingly function as clinicians of first contact. Nurse practitioners also play an indispensable clinical role in large HMOs and disease management companies. Nurses are drawn to primary care roles in increasing numbers, but we are likely to face significant future problems in meeting nursing needs in hospitals and nursing homes, and large shortages are forecast.

Although the public has a high opinion of nurses, nurses continue to have less status than other professional groups. Many women who in the past opted for nursing careers now enter other professions, including medicine, business, and law. Many within nursing seek more independent and prestigious roles as nurse practitioners and nurse specialists. Hospitals, the largest users of general nursing services, face recruitment problems and tough competition. Nurses who work in hospitals have less control over their work and less autonomy than those who pursue more independent roles. Hospital nursing is particularly demanding work, both mentally and physically. Work stress has increased as hospitals have much sicker caseloads than in prior times, and nurses have more intensive responsibilities. Faced with reimbursement pressures, hospitals have reduced nursing staff, increasing the stresses and workload for those who remain. Studies show that lower nurse-to-patient ratios in hospitals result in lower-quality care and increased patient mortality, as well as nurse dissatisfaction and burnout.[10] To make matters worse, nurses still often have poor relationships with physicians and feel that their contributions and expertise are not valued. Many of these nurses aspire to leave hospital nursing.

Nursing organizations have sought aggressively to have states mandate minimum nurse-to-patient requirements in hospitals. California was the first state to mandate such ratios; California hospitals strongly opposed them, arguing that such mandates exacerbate the nursing shortage. The legislation, first passed in 1999, had a staged process for putting required ratios into place. Since January 2004, hospitals were required to have one nurse for every six patients in medical/surgical units. This was scheduled to increase to one for every five patients in January 2005. In response to hospital pressures, Governor Arnold Schwarzenegger attempted to freeze implementation through an emergency regulation vigorously opposed by California nurses, who succeeded in blocking his attempt. In March 2005, the California Superior Court reinstated the minimum one nurse to every five patients in medical/surgical units. Similar efforts to introduce minimum nurse-staffing ratios are being pursued in other states. Nurses have built a strong case for more intense staffing based on the safety issue and the link between nurse staffing and patient outcomes.

Hospital administrators have adapted to difficulty in recruiting nurses by increasing salaries, allowing nurses to work in three-day, twelve-hour shifts, and showing a bit more flexibility in other work conditions. But the increasing severity of illness among hospital patients and reduced staffing combine to make the hospital nursing experience more frantic and difficult than it was in the past. Hospitals facing recruitment difficulties often fill in by using agency nurses, rotating nurses among services depending upon need, and making other management decisions that treat nursing more as a general utility service than as a profession. Such solutions harm continuity of care, make it likely that nurses will be unfamiliar with unit procedures, create social distance between nurses and doctors, who increasingly don't know each other, and probably contribute to hospital error and patient injury as well. The hospital nursing workforce is increasing in average age. Without significant changes that attract more young recruits, hospital nurse shortages are likely to become a major problem. Hospitals aggressively recruit foreign nurses, thus depleting systems far more needy than our own and exacerbating language and cultural problems in American hospitals.

There are literally hundreds of issues important to the future of our health care system and ultimately our health. Those that elicit some of the greatest professional passions and public attention, such as the issues of malpractice litigation and physician payment, are not necessarily those that are most important. Many of the seemingly more boring and technical issues, to which the public does not much attend, have greater import; these include such issues as disseminating appropriate information technology and adapting legal frameworks more consistent with evolving medical science, technology, and ethics. The legal framework of health care, including issues relating to managing competition, restraint of trade, managed care, privacy, ethical research, and patients' rights, is a quiet hand that importantly shapes care provision and costs. Even the malpractice issue, which receives much media attention, is typically focused on malpractice insurance costs and rarely on the more central and important question of what kind of system is fair to providers, equitable for patients, that properly and reliably compensates persons who are injured through negligence.

Medical systems are complicated, but organizing and providing quality care is not rocket science. Most necessary care, most of the time, is very basic and can be handled expeditiously, efficiently, and without enormous expense. The cost of extending health coverage to the forty-six million people now uninsured and guaranteeing a system that is universal for all is clearly within our technical and economic capability. We can claim that medical technology in the United States is second to none, but we offer citizens a mediocre system that is below reasonable expectations in maintaining health, preventing disease, and providing ready access to treatment for many once they become ill. American health care is not only not the best, as we like to brag; it is too often an embarrassment. Failure to overcome our health system dysfunctions is not a result of lack of knowledge or organizational capacity. It is an issue of will and commitment. At some point, we as a nation will have to decide whether we wish to design our health care system primarily to satisfy those who profit from it or to protect the health and welfare of all Americans. No one promises that achieving universal or higher quality health care will be easy or even that they are inevitable. But anything is possible if the public begins to appreciate how little it gets for what it really pays and organizes politically to promote a health care system that is fairer, more inclusive, and offers more value for money.

Notes

Introduction

1. Henry A. Waxman, "The Lessons of Vioxx—Drug Safety and Sales," *New England Journal of Medicine* 352, no. 25 (June 23, 2005): 2576–2578.

2. Alex Berenson, "At Vioxx Trial, A Discrepancy Appears to Undercut Merck's Defense," *New York Times*, July 20, 2005, C1 and C9.

3. Debabrata Mukherjee, Steven E. Nissen, and Eric J. Topol, "Risk of Cardiovascular Events Associated with Selective Cox-2 Inhibitors," *Journal of the American Medical Association* 286, no. 8 (August 22/29, 2001): 954–959.

4. Eric J. Topol, "Arthritis Medicines and Cardiovascular Events—'House of Coxibs,'" *Journal of the American Medical Association* 293, no. 3 (January 19, 2005): 366–368.

5. Robert Steinbrook, "The Controversy Over Guidant's Implantable Defibrillators," *New England Journal of Medicine* 353, no. 3 (July 21, 2005): 221–224.

6. See Keith Wailoo, *Drawing Blood: Technology and Disease Identity in Twentieth-Century America* (Baltimore, Md.: Johns Hopkins University Press, 1997).

7. Rosemary A. Stevens, *American Medicine and the Public Interest*, updated ed. (Berkeley: University of California Press, 1998).

8. Sheila M. Rothman and David J. Rothman, *The Pursuit of Perfection: The Promise and Perils of Medical Enhancement* (New York: Pantheon Books, 2003); Carl Elliott, *Better Than Well: American Medicine Meets the American Dream* (New York: W. W. Norton, 2003).

9. David Mechanic, "The Rise and Fall of Managed Care," *Journal of Health and Social Behavior* 45, extra issue (December 2004): 76–86.

10. Families USA, *One in Three: Non-Elderly Americans Without Health Insurance, 2002–2003*. Publication No. 04-104, June 2004. Available online: www.familiesusa.org.

11. Gerard F. Anderson, Peter S. Hussey, Bianca K. Frogner, and Hugh R. Waters, "Health Spending in the United States and the Rest of the Industrialized World," *Health Affairs* 24, no. 4 (July/August 2005): 903–914.

12. Brian D. Smedley, Adrienne Y. Stith, and Alan R. Nelson, eds., *Unequal Treatment: Confronting Racial and Ethnic Disparities in Health Care* (Washington, D.C.: National Academies Press, 2003).

13. The SUPPORT Principal Investigators, "A Controlled Trial to Improve Care for Seriously Ill Hospitalized Patients," *Journal of the American Medical Association* 274, no. 20 (November 22–29, 1995): 1591–1598.

14. Linda T. Kohn, Janet M. Corrigan, and Molla S. Donaldson, eds., *To Err Is Human: Building a Safer Health System* (Washington, D.C.: National Academies Press, 2000).

15. Lucian L. Leape, "Preventing Medical Errors," in *Policy Challenges in Modern Health Care*, ed. David Mechanic, Lynn B. Rogut, David C. Colby, and James R. Knickman (New Brunswick, N.J.: Rutgers University Press, 2005), 162–176.

16. Michael T. Osterholm, "Preparing for the Next Pandemic," *New England Journal of Medicine* 352, no. 18 (May 5, 2005): 1839–1842.

17. Dennis Normile, "Genetic Analyses Suggest Bird Flu Virus Is Evolving," *Science* 308, no. 5726 (May 27, 2005): 1234–1235.

18. Robert Masterton, "Antibiotic Resistance in Nosocomial Infections." Available online: www.infectionacademy.org.

Chapter 1 — Is Reform Possible?

1. [Institute of Medicine, Committee on Pain, Disability, and Chronic Illness Behavior] Marian Osterweis, Arthur Kleinman, and David Mechanic, eds., *Pain and Disability: Clinical, Behavioral and Public Policy Perspectives* (Washington, D.C.: National Academies Press, 1987).

2. Richard A. Deyo, Alf Nachemson, and Sohail K. Mirza, "Spinal-Fusion Surgery— The Case for Restraint," *New England Journal of Medicine* 350, no. 7 (February 12, 2004): 722–726.

3. Richard A. Deyo, Bruce M. Psaty, Gregory Simon, et al., "The Messenger Under Attack—Intimidation of Researchers by Special Interest Groups," *New England Journal of Medicine* 336, no. 16 (April 17, 1997): 1176–1180.

4. John K. Iglehart, "Health Policy Report: Politics and Public Health," *New England Journal of Medicine* 334, no. 3 (January 18, 1996): 203–207.

5. Mark R. Chassin and Elise C. Becher, "The Wrong Patient," *Annals of Internal Medicine* 136, no. 11 (June 4, 2002): 826–833.

6. For a detailed analysis of the managed care backlash, see Mechanic, "The Rise and Fall of Managed Care" (see note 9, introduction).

7. John Holahan and Allison Cook, "Changes in Economic Conditions and Health Insurance Coverage, 2000–2004," *Health Affairs Web Exclusive,* November 2005. Available online: http://content.healthaffairs.org. Also see Institute of Medicine, *Insuring America's Health: Principles and Recommendations* (Washington, D.C.: National Academies Press, 2004).

8. Institute of Medicine, *Care without Coverage: Too Little, Too Late* (Washington, D.C.: National Academies Press, 2002). Although selection factors are difficult to fully control for, the Institute of Medicine reports that the risk of death resulting from lack of insurance may be as much as one-quarter to one-third higher than among those who are insured.

9. Cathy Schoen, Michelle M. Doty, Sara R. Collins, et al., "Insured But Not Protected: How Many Adults Are Underinsured?" *Health Affairs Web Exclusive*, June 14, 2005. Available online: http://content.healthaffairs.org. The researchers in this study defined underinsurance as having medical expenses equal to 10 percent or more of income or, in the case of the poor, 5 percent of income, or having plan deductibles of at least 5 percent of income.

10. Stephen Heffler, Sheila Smith, Sean Keehan, et al. "Health Spending Projections For 2002–2012," *Health Affairs Web Exclusive*, February 7, 2003. Available online: http://content.healthaffairs.org.

11. William B. Schwartz, *Life without Disease: The Pursuit of Medical Utopia* (Berkeley: University of California Press, 1998); also see David M. Cutler, *Your Money or Your Life: Strong Medicine for America's Health Care System* (New York: Oxford University Press, 2004), for a discussion of the increasing value of medical care.

12. William C. Black and H. Gilbert Welch, "Advances in Diagnostic Imaging and Overestimations of Disease Prevalence and the Benefits of Therapy," *New England Journal of Medicine* 328, no. 17 (April 29, 1993): 1237–1243.

13. Elliott S. Fisher and H. Gilbert Welch, "Avoiding the Unintended Consequences of Growth in Medical Care: How Might More Be Worse?" *Journal of the American Medical Association* 281, no. 5 (February 3, 1999): 446–453.

14. Ibid.

15. Abraham B. Bergman and Stanley J. Stamm, "The Morbidity of Cardiac Nondisease in Schoolchildren," *New England Journal of Medicine* 276, no. 18 (May 4, 1967): 1008–1013.

16. Fisher and Welch, "Avoiding the Unintended Consequences of Growth in Medical Care," 449.

17. Richard A. Deyo and Donald L. Patrick, *Hope or Hype: The Obsession with Medical Advances and the High Cost of False Promises* (New York: AMACOM, 2005).

18. Ole Olsen and Peter C. Gøtzsche, "Cochrane Review on Screening for Breast Cancer with Mammography," *The Lancet* 358, no. 9290 (October 20, 2001): 1340–1342.

19. Elizabeth A. McGlynn, Steven M. Asch, John Adams, et al., "The Quality of Health Care Delivered to Adults in the United States," *New England Journal of Medicine* 348, no. 26 (June 26, 2003): 2635–2645.

20. Paul Starr, *The Social Transformation of American Medicine* (New York: Basic Books, 1982); Jill Quadagno, *One Nation Uninsured: Why the U.S. Has No National Health Insurance* (New York: Oxford University Press, 2005); Colin Gordon, *Dead on Arrival: The Politics of Health Care in Twentieth-Century America* (Princeton, N.J.: Princeton University Press, 2003); Alan Derickson, *Health Security For All: Dreams of Universal Health Care in America* (Baltimore, Md.: Johns Hopkins University Press, 2005); for a political economy perspective, see Sherry Glied, *Chronic Condition: Why Health Reform Fails* (Cambridge: Harvard University Press, 1997); for a more general discussion, see Seymour Martin Lipset, *American Exceptionalism: A Double-Edged Sword* (New York: W. W. Norton, 1996).

21. Mechanic, "The Rise and Fall of Managed Care."

22. Robert H. Miller and Harold S. Luft, "Does Managed Care Lead to Better or Worse Quality of Care?" *Health Affairs* 16, no. 5 (September/October 1997): 7–25; "HMO Plan Performance Update: An Analysis of the Literature, 1997–2001," *Health Affairs* 21, no. 4 (July/August 2002): 63–86.

23. Glen P. Mays, Gary Claxton, and Justin White, "Managed Care Rebound? Recent Changes in Health Plans' Cost Containment Strategies," *Health Affairs Web Exclusive*, August 11, 2004. Available online: http://content.healthaffairs.org.

24. James A. Morone, *Hellfire Nation: The Politics of Sin in American History* (New Haven, Conn.: Yale University Press, 2003).

25. John Sheils and Randall Haught, "The Cost of Tax-Exempt Health Benefits in 2004," *Health Affairs Web Exclusive*, February 25, 2004. Available online: http://content.healthaffairs.org.

26. John Sheils and Paul Hogan, "Cost of Tax-Exempt Health Benefits in 1998," *Health Affairs* 18, no. 2 (March/April 1999): 176–181.

27. Sheils and Haught, "The Cost of Tax-Exempt Health Benefits."

28. Scott C. Williams, Stephen P. Schmaltz, David J. Morton, et al., "Quality of Care in U.S. Hospitals as Reflected by Standardized Measures, 2002–2004," *New England Journal of Medicine* 353, no. 3 (July 21, 2005): 255–264.

29. Patrick S. Romano, "Improving the Quality of Hospital Care in America," *New England Journal of Medicine* 353, no. 3 (July 21, 2005): 302–304.

30. Judith H. Hibbard, Jean Stockard, and Martin Tusler, "Hospital Performance Reports: Impact on Quality, Market Share, and Reputation," *Health Affairs* 24, no. 4 (July/August 2005): 1150–1160.

31. See Jerome P. Kassirer, *On the Take: How Medicine's Complicity With Big Business Can Endanger Your Health* (New York: Oxford University Press, 2005).

32. Deyo et al., "The Messenger Under Attack," 1176–1180.

33. The Henry J. Kaiser Family Foundation/Agency for Healthcare Research and Quality. *National Survey on Americans as Health Care Consumers: An Update on the Role of Quality Information*. December 2000. Available online: http://www.kff.org.

34. Norman Daniels and James E. Sabin, *Setting Limits Fairly: Can We Learn to Share Medical Resources?* (New York: Oxford University Press, 2002).

35. George C. Halvorson and George J. Isham, *Epidemic of Care: A Call for Safer, Better and More Accountable Health Care* (San Francisco: Jossey-Bass, 2003).

36. McGlynn et al., "The Quality of Health Care Delivered to Adults," 2635–2645.

37. Kohn et al., *To Err Is Human* (see note 14, introduction).

38. David Mechanic, "The Functions and Limitations of Trust in the Provision of Medical Care," *Journal of Health Politics, Policy and Law* 23, no. 4 (August 1998): 661–686.

39. Robert R. Alford, *Health Care Politics: Ideological and Interest Group Barriers to Reform* (Chicago: University of Chicago Press, 1975).

40. Carol S. Weissert and William G. Weissert, *Governing Health: The Politics of Health Policy*, 2nd ed. (Baltimore, Md.: Johns Hopkins University Press, 2002).

41. James C. Robinson, *The Corporate Practice of Medicine: Competition and Innovation in Health Care* (Berkeley: University of California Press, 1999).

Chapter 2 — What Is Disease and What Should We Treat?

1. Avshalom Caspi, Karen Sugden, Terrie E. Moffitt, et al., "Influence of Life Stress on Depression: Moderation by a Polymorphism in the 5-HTT Gene," *Science* 301, no. 5631 (July 18, 2003): 386–389.

2. David Mechanic, *Medical Sociology*, 2nd ed. (New York: Free Press, 1978), 95–99.

3. René J. Dubos, *Mirage of Health: Utopias, Progress and Biological Change*, (1959; reprint, New Brunswick, N.J.: Rutgers University Press, 1987), 38–39.

4. Neil C. Campbell and Peter Murchie, "Treating Hypertension with Guidelines in General Practice," *British Medical Journal* 329, no. 7465 (September 4, 2004): 523–524.

5. Ramachandran S. Vasan, Alexa Beiser, Sudha Seshadri, et al., "Residual Lifetime Risk for Developing Hypertension in Middle-Aged Women and Men: The Framingham Heart Study," *Journal of the American Medical Association* 287, no. 8 (February 27, 2002): 1003–1010.

6. Nicholas J. Wald and Malcolm R Law, "A Strategy to Reduce Cardiovascular Disease by More than 80%," *British Medical Journal* 326, no. 7404 (June 28, 2003): 1419–1423.

7. Osterweis et al., *Pain and Disability* (see note 1, chapter 1), 193–205.

8. Henry K. Beecher, *Measurement of Subjective Responses: Quantitative Effects of Drugs* (New York: Oxford University Press, 1959).

9. Kerr L. White, T. Franklin Williams, and Bernard G. Greenberg, "The Ecology of Medical Care," *New England Journal of Medicine* 265, no. 18 (November 2, 1961): 885–892.

10. David Mechanic and Margaret Newton, "Some Problems in the Analysis of Morbidity Data," *Journal of Chronic Diseases* 18 (June 1965): 569–580.

11. Larry A. Green, George E. Fryer Jr., Barbara P. Yawn, et al., "The Ecology of Medical Care Revisited," *New England Journal of Medicine* 344, no. 26 (June 28, 2001): 2021–2025.

12. David Mechanic and Ronald J. Angel, "Some Factors Associated with the Report and Evaluation of Back Pain," *Journal of Health and Social Behavior* 28, no. 2 (June 1987): 131–139.

13. Joseph P. Newhouse and the Insurance Experiment Group, *Free For All?: Lessons from the RAND Health Insurance Experiment* (Cambridge: Harvard University Press, 1993).

14. Michael L. Millenson, *Demanding Medical Excellence: Doctors and Accountability in the Information Age* (Chicago: University of Chicago Press, 1997).

15. David Mechanic, "Is the Prevalence of Mental Disorders a Good Measure of the Need for Services?" *Health Affairs* 22, no. 5 (September/October 2003): 8–20.

16. Ronald C. Kessler, Patricia Berglund, Olga Demler, et al., "The Epidemiology of Major Depressive Disorder: Results from the National Comorbidity Survey Replication (NCS-R)," *Journal of the American Medical Association* 289, no. 23 (June 18, 2003): 3095–3105.

Chapter 3 — Saving Lives Individually or in Populations

1. Robert Evans, *Interpreting and Addressing Inequality in Health: From Black to Acheson to Blair to . . . ?* (London: Office of Health Economics, 2002).

2. Gerald N. Grob, *The Deadly Truth: A History of Disease in America* (Cambridge: Harvard University Press, 2002).

3. Cutler, *Your Money or Your Life* (see note 11, chapter 1).

4. Jeannette A. Rogowski, Douglas O. Staiger, and Jeffrey D. Horbar, "Variations in the Quality of Care for Very-Low-Birthweight Infants: Implications for Policy," *Health Affairs* 23, no. 5 (September/October 2004): 88–97.

5. Maureen Hack, H. Gerry Taylor, Dennis Drotar, et al., "Chronic Conditions, Functional Limitations, and Special Health Care Needs of School-aged Children Born with Extremely Low-Birth-Weight in the 1990s," *Journal of the American Medical Association* 294, no. 3 (July 20, 2005): 318–325.

6. To see an example of contradictions between theory and data, see Reuel A. Stallones, "The Rise and Fall of Ischemic Heart Disease," *Scientific American* 243, no. 5 (November 1980): 53–59; for a discussion of role of cardiovascular technology, see Cutler, *Your Money or Your Life.*

7. Ali H. Mokdad, James S. Marks, Donna F. Stroup, et al., "Actual Causes of Death in the United States, 2000," *Journal of the American Medical Association* 291, no. 10 (March 10, 2004): 1238–1245; also see J. Michael McGinnis and William H. Foege, "Actual Causes of Deaths in the United States," *Journal of the American Medical Association* 270, no. 18 (November 10, 1993): 2207–2212.

8. Geoffrey Rose, "Sick Individuals and Sick Populations," *International Journal of Epidemiology* 14, no. 1 (March 1985): 32–38.

9. Ibid.

10. Sir Donald Acheson, *Independent Inquiry into Inequalities in Health: Report* (London: The Stationery Office, 1998); Michaela Benzeval, Ken Judge, and Margaret Whitehead, *Tackling Inequalities in Health: An Agenda for Action* (London: The King's Fund, 1995).

11. This literature is very extensive. For a brief review, see David Mechanic, "Rediscovering the Social Determinants of Health," *Health Affairs* 19, no. 3 (May/June 2000): 269–276. Some useful collections include John P. Bunker, Deanna S. Gomby, and Barbara H. Kehrer, eds., *Pathways to Health: The Role of Social Factors* (Menlo Park, Calif.: Henry J. Kaiser Family Foundation, 1989); George Davey Smith, ed., *Health Inequalities: Lifecourse Approaches* (Bristol, UK: Policy Press, 2003); Ichiro Kawachi, Bruce P. Kennedy, and Richard G. Wilkinson, eds., *The Society and Population Health Reader*, vol. 1, *Income Inequality and Health* (New York: The New Press, 1999).

12. Aaron Antonovsky, "Social Class, Life Expectancy and Overall Mortality," *Milbank Quarterly* 45, no. 2 (April 1967): 31–73.
13. Some examples include Evelyn M. Kitagawa and Philip M. Hauser, *Differential Mortality in the United States: A Study in Socioeconomic Epidemiology* (Cambridge: Harvard University Press, 1973); Ronald C. Kessler, "A Disaggregation of the Relationship Between Socioeconomic Status and Psychological Distress," *American Sociological Review* 47, no. 6 (December 1982): 752–764.
14. David R. Williams, "Patterns and Causes of Disparities in Health" in Mechanic et al., *Policy Challenges* (see note 15, introduction), 115–134.
15. John Lynch, George Davey Smith, Sam Harper, et al., "Is Income Inequality a Determinant of Population Health? Part I: A Systematic Review," *Milbank Quarterly* 82, no. 1 (March 2004): 5–99; also see Smith, *Health Inequalities*.
16. Bruce G. Link and Jo Phelan, "Social Conditions as Fundamental Causes of Disease," *Journal of Health and Social Behavior* (Extra Issue 1995): 80–94; also see Bruce G. Link and Jo C. Phelan, "Fundamental Sources of Health Inequalities" in Mechanic et al., *Policy Challenges* (see note 15, introduction), 71–84.
17. There have been many publications based on the Whitehall studies. Some representative papers include Michael G. Marmot, Martin J. Shipley, and Geoffrey Rose, "Inequalities in Death-Specific Explanations of a General Pattern?" *The Lancet* 323, no. 8384 (May 5, 1984): 1003–1006; Michael G. Marmot and Martin J. Shipley, "Do Socioeconomic Differences in Mortality Persist After Retirement? Twenty-Five Year Follow-up of Civil Servants from the First Whitehall Study," *British Medical Journal* 313, no. 7066 (November 9, 1996): 1177–1180.
18. Richard G. Wilkinson, "Putting the Picture Together: Prosperity, Redistribution, Health and Welfare," in *Social Determinants of Health*, ed. Michael Marmot and Richard G. Wilkinson (Oxford: Oxford University Press, 1999) 256–274; and Eric Brunner and Michael Marmot, "Social Organization, Stress, and Health," in Marmot and Wilkinson, *Social Determinants of Health*, 17–43. For a more general review, see Michael G. Marmot, *The Status Syndrome: How Social Standing Affects our Health and Longevity* (New York: Times Books, 2004).
19. Ichiro Kawachi and Bruce P. Kennedy, *The Health of Nations: Why Inequality Is Harmful to Your Health* (New York: The New Press, 2002), and Kawachi, Kennedy, and Wilkinson, *The Society and Population Health Reader*, vol. 1, *Income Inequality and Health*.
20. For an excellent review of the research literature, see Lynch et al., "Is Income Inequality a Determinant of Population Health?" 5–99.
21. Angus Deaton and Darren Lubotsky, "Mortality, Inequality and Race in American Cities and States," *Social Science and Medicine* 56, no. 6 (March 2003): 1139–1153. Also see Jennifer M. Mellor and Jeffrey Milyo, "Reexamining the Evidence of an Ecological Association Between Income Inequality and Health," *Journal of Health Politics, Policy and Law* 26, no. 3 (June 2001): 487–522.
22. Dominance hierarchies have a range of physiological and health effects in many species but the patterns are complex and vary. See Robert M. Sapolsky, "The Influence of Social Hierarchy on Primate Health," *Science* 308, no. 5722 (April 29, 2005): 648–652; also see Robert M. Sapolsky, *Why Zebras Don't Get Ulcers*, 3rd ed. (New York: Henry Holt , 2004).
23. Richard G. Wilkinson, "Social Relations, Hierarchy, and Health," in *The Society and Population Health Reader*, vol. 2, *A State and Community Perspective*, ed. Alvin R. Tarlov and Robert F. St. Peter (New York: The New Press, 1999) 205–229.

24. For an excellent review of this literature, see [Committee on Understanding and Eliminating Racial and Ethnic Disparities in Health Care, Board on Health Sciences Policy, Institute of Medicine] Brian D. Smedley, Adrienne Y. Stith and Alan R. Nelson, eds., *Unequal Treatment: Confronting Racial and Ethnic Disparities in Health Care* (Washington, D.C.: National Academies Press, 2003).

25. There is a seemingly paradoxical finding that some poor Hispanic populations in the United States such as Mexican Americans have better mortality experiences than the native-born white population. There are many efforts to understand the basis of the "Hispanic paradox," and some believe that selection effects are an important explanation for this finding. See Alberto Palloni and Jeffrey D. Morenoff, "Interpreting the Paradoxical in the Hispanic Paradox: Demographic and Epidemiological Approaches," *Annals of the New York Academy of Sciences* 954, no. 1 (December 2001): 140–174.

26. Rubén G. Rumbaut, "Origins and Destinies: Immigration, Race, and Ethnicity in Contemporary America," in *Origins and Destinies: Immigration, Race and Ethnicity in America*, ed. Silvia Pedraza and Rubén G. Rumbaut (Belmont, Calif.: Wadsworth, 1996) 21–42.

27. Alejandro Portes and Rubén G. Rumbaut, *Legacies: The Story of the Immigrant Second Generation* (Berkeley: University of California Press, 2001).

28. Williams, *Policy Challenges in Modern Health Care*, 115–134; Jen'nan Ghazal Read, Michael O. Emerson, and Alvin Tarlov, "Implications of Black Immigrant Health for U.S. Racial Disparities in Health," *Journal of Immigrant Health* 7, no. 3 (July 2005): 205–212.

29. Peter Bach, Hoangmai H. Pham, Deborah Schrag, et al., "Primary Care Physicians Who Treat Blacks and Whites," *New England Journal of Medicine* 351, no. 6 (August 5, 2004): 575–584; also see Smedley et al., *Unequal Treatment*.

30. David Mechanic, "Disadvantage, Inequality and Social Policy," *Health Affairs* 21, no. 2 (March/April 2002): 48–59.

31. Kenneth E. Warner, "The Need for, and Value of, A Multi-Level Approach to Disease Prevention: The Case of Tobacco Control," in Committee on Capitalizing on Social Science and Behavioral Research to Improve the Public's Health, *Promoting Health: Intervention Strategies From Social and Behavioral Research*, ed. Brian D. Smedley and S. Leonard Syme (Washington, D.C.: National Academies Press, 2000) 417–449; Kenneth E. Warner, "Tobacco Policy in the United States: Lessons for the Obesity Epidemic," in Mechanic et al., *Policy Challenges* (see note 15, introduction), 99–114.

32. For a fascinating history of lead and related environmental threats, see Gerald Markowitz and David Rosner, *Deceit and Denial: The Deadly Politics of Industrial Pollution* (Berkeley: University of California Press, 2002).

33. Robert D. Putnam, *Bowling Alone: The Collapse and Revival of American Community* (New York: Simon and Schuster, 2000); James S. Coleman, *Foundations of Social Theory* (Cambridge: Belknap Press of Harvard University Press, 1990).

34. See John C. Caldwell, "Routes to Low Mortality in Poor Countries," *Population and Development Review* 12, no. 2 (June 1986): 171–220); Deon Filmer and Lant Pritchett, "The Impact of Public Spending on Health: Does Money Matter?" *Social Science and Medicine* 49, no. 10 (November 1999): 1309–1323.

35. Reed Geertsen, Melville R. Klauber, Mark Rindflesh, et al., "A Re-Examination of Suchman's Views on Social Factors in Health Care Utilization," *Journal of Health and Social Behavior* 16, no. 2 (June 1975): 226–237.

36. Thomas F. O'Dea, *The Mormons* (Chicago: University of Chicago Press, 1957).

37. In a classic discussion, Victor Fuchs, *Who Shall Live?: Health, Economics, and Social Choice* (New York: Basic Books, 1974), includes a section (pages 52–55) entitled "A Tale of Two States" in which he compares disease and mortality rates in Nevada and Utah, states that are contiguous and have comparable levels of medical care and economic conditions. However, health levels in these two states vary enormously, which Fuchs links to their vastly different cultures and lifestyles.

38. James A. Morone, *Hellfire Nation: The Politics of Sin in American History* (New Haven, Conn.: Yale University Press, 2003).

Chapter 4 — The Murky Challenge of Mental Health

1. Tami Mark, Rosanna M. Coffey, David McKusick, et al., *National Estimates of Expenditures for Mental Health Services and Substance Abuse Treatment, 1991–2001*, SAMHSA publication no. SMA 05-3999 (Rockville, Md.: Substance Abuse and Mental Health Services Administration, 2005).

2. Rick Mayes and Allan Horwitz, "DSM-III and the Revolution in the Classification of Mental Illness," *Journal of History of the Behavioral Sciences* 41, no. 3 (Summer 2005): 249–267.

3. Philip S. Wang, Michael Lane, Mark Olfson, et al., "Twelve-Month Use of Mental Health Services in the United States," *Archives of General Psychiatry* 62, no. 6 (June 2005): 629–640.

4. Gerald N. Grob, *The Mad Among Us: A History of the Care of America's Mentally Ill* (New York: Free Press, 1994).

5. David Mechanic, *Mental Health and Social Policy: The Emergence of Managed Care*, 4th ed. (Boston: Allyn and Bacon, 1999).

6. A program of training for primary care physicians called Balint groups was built around analyzing these situations. These efforts were named for Michael Balint, *The Doctor, His Patient and the Illness* (New York: International Universities Press, 1957).

7. For an interesting history of this issue, see Edward Shorter, *From Paralysis to Fatigue: A History of Psychosomatic Illness in the Modern Era* (New York: Free Press, 1992), and Edward Shorter, *From the Mind Into the Body: The Cultural Origins of Psychosomatic Symptoms* (New York: Free Press, 1994); also see Arthur Kleinman, *Social Origins of Distress and Disease: Depression, Neurasthenia, and Pain in Modern China* (New Haven, Conn.: Yale University Press, 1986).

8. There is a large literature on these patterns, for example, Norman Sartorius, David Goldberg, Giovanni de Girolamo, et al., eds., *Psychological Disorders in General Medical Settings* (Toronto: Hogrefe and Huber, 1990).

9. Mechanic, *Medical Sociology* (see note 2, chapter 2).

10. Ellen L. Idler and Yael Benyamini, "Self-Rated Health and Mortality: A Review of Twenty-Seven Community Studies," *Journal of Health and Social Behavior* 38, no. 1 (March 1997): 21–37.

11. The major sources of these estimates have been the Epidemiological Catchment Area (ECA) Study and the National Comorbidity Study (NCS). See Lee N. Robins and Darrel A. Regier, eds., *Psychiatric Disorders in America: The Epidemiological Catchment Area Study* (New York: Free Press, 1991), and Ronald C. Kessler, Katherine A. McGonagle, Shanyang Zhao, et al., "Lifetime and 12-month Prevalence of DSM-III-R Psychiatric Disorders in the United States: Results From the National Comorbidity Study," *Archives of General Psychiatry* 51, no. 1 (January 1994): 8–19.

More recent reports from the National Comorbidity Survey Replication include Ronald C. Kessler, Wai Tat Chiu, Olga Demler, et al., "Prevalence, Severity and Comorbidity of 12-Month DSM-IV Disorders in the National Comorbidity Survey Replication," *Archives of General Psychiatry* 62, no. 6 (June 2005): 617–627; Philip S. Wang, Patricia Berglund, Mark Olfson, et al., "Failure and Delay in Initial Treatment Contact After First Onset of Mental Disorders in the National Comorbidity Survey Replication," *Archives of General Psychiatry* 62, no. 6 (June 2005): 603–613; and Wang et al., "Twelve-Month Use of Mental Health Services in the United States," 629–640.

12. Mechanic, "Is the Prevalence of Mental Disorders a Good Measure of the Need for Services?" (see note 15, chapter 2).

13. For an example, see William E. Narrow, Donald S. Rae, Lee N. Robins, et al., "Revised Prevalence Estimates of Mental Disorders in the United States: Using A Clinical Significance Criterion to Reconcile 2 Surveys' Estimates," *Archives of General Psychiatry* 59, no. 2 (February 2002): 115–123. Using questions about life interference, telling a professional about one's symptoms, or using medication, these authors report prevalence estimates 17 percent lower than in the ECA studies and 32 percent lower than in the NCS.

14. Jerome C. Wakefield and Robert L. Spitzer, "Lowered Estimates—But of What?" *Archives of General Psychiatry* 59, no. 2 (February 2002): 129–130.

15. For an example of such efforts, see Ronald C. Kessler, Patricia A. Berglund, Shanyang Zhao, Philip J. Leaf, et al., "The 12-Month Prevalence and Correlates of Serious Mental Illness (SMI)" in *Mental Health, United States, 1996*, ed. Ronald W. Manderscheid and Mary Anne Sonnenschein,. 59–70, DHHS pub. no. (SMA) 96-3098 (Washington, D.C.: U.S. Government Printing Office, 1996).

16. A recent analysis [Philip S. Wang, Patricia A. Berglund, Mark Olfson, et al., "Delays in Initial Treatment Contact After First Onset of a Mental Disorder," *Health Services Research* 39, no. 2 (April 2004): 393–415] found that 80 percent of people who reached criteria for a disorder at some point in their lives eventually received some form of treatment. Those with more severe indications received treatment earlier, but delays were long; in the case of depression median delay was seven years.

17. Wang et al., "Twelve-Month Use of Mental Health Services in the United States," 629–640.

18. U.S. Department of Health and Human Services, *Evalution of Parity in the Federal Employees Health Benefits (FEHB) Program*, Final Report, December 2004.

19. Mechanic, *Mental Health and Social Policy*.

20. David Mechanic, "Managing Behavioral Health in Medicaid," *New England Journal of Medicine* 348, no. 19 (May 8, 2003): 1914–1916.

21. See Anthony F. Lehman, "Quality of Care in Mental Health: The Case of Schizophrenia," *Health Affairs* 18, no. 5 (September/October 1999): 52–65; Ronald C. Kessler, Patricia Berglund, Olga Demler, et al., "The Epidemiology of Major Depressive Disorder: Results From the National Comorbidity Survey Replication (NCS-R), *Journal of the American Medical Association* 289, no. 23 (June 18, 2003): 3095–3105.

22. David Mechanic and Donna D. McAlpine, "Mission Unfulfilled: Potholes on the Road to Mental Health Parity" *Health Affairs* 18, no. 5 (September/October 1999): 7–21.

23. David Mechanic and Scott Bilder, "Treatment of People with Mental Illness: A Decade-Long Perspective," *Health Affairs* 23, no. 4 (July/August 2004): 84–95.

24. Wang et al., "Twelve-Month Use of Mental Health Services in the United States," 629–640.

25. Olfson and colleagues found in analyzing data from the National Ambulatory Medical Care Survey that treatment for depression increased threefold from 1987 to 1997. Most of those treated received SSRIs. Mark Olfson, Steven C. Marcus, Benjamin Druss, et al., "National Trends in the Outpatient Treatment of Depression," *Journal of the American Medical Association* 287, no. 2 (January 9, 2002): 203–209.

26. Many clinicians argue for the superiority of combination therapy, but the research evidence remains weak, particularly in reference to adolescents and children. Thus, much excitement and media attention greeted a recent publication in the *Journal of the American Medical Association* by the Treatment for Adolescents with Depression Study Team: "Fluoxetine, Cognitive-Behavioral Therapy, and Their Combination for Adolescents with Depression: Treatment for Adolescents with Depression Study (TADS) Randomized Controlled Trial," *Journal of the American Medical Association* 292, no. 7 (August 18, 2004): 807–820, that found 71 percent receiving combination therapy improved over a twelve-week intervention compared with 60 percent for those treated with fluoxetine alone, 43 percent with cognitive behavioral therapy alone, and 35 percent placebo. The paper acknowledged the serious problem of the combination group not being blinded as compared to the fluoxetine group, with the possibility that the 11 percent difference in results could be accounted for by the nonblinded expectancy effects, but press releases and media coverage failed to make this limitation apparent. For an excellent critique of the media coverage, see Jeanne Lenzer, "Journalists on Prozac: Did Major Media Outlets Fail To Ask the Right Questions About Depression Study?" *British Medical Journal* 329, no. 7468 (September 25, 2004): 748.

27. Joanna Moncrieff and Irving Kirsch, "Efficacy of Antidepressants in Adults," *British Medical Journal* 331, no. 7509 (16 July 2005): 155–157.

28. Kenneth B. Wells, Roland Sturm, Cathy D. Sherbourne, et al., *Caring for Depression* (Cambridge: Harvard University Press, 1996).

29. Kenneth B. Wells and his colleagues, in a randomized intervention program directed to a diverse group of managed primary care settings, demonstrated that quality of depression care and outcomes can be improved over a year. Kenneth B. Wells, Cathy Sherbourne, Michael Schoenbaum, et al., "Impact of Disseminating Quality Improvement Programs for Depression in Managed Primary Care: A Randomized Controlled Trial," *Journal of the American Medical Association* 283, no. 2 (January 12, 2000): 212–220. A subsequent cost-effectiveness analysis found that the benefits relative to costs were comparable to the results found with accepted medical interventions in terms of costs per quality adjusted life year. See Michael Schoenbaum, Jürgen Unützer, Cathy Sherbourne, et al., "Cost-Effectiveness of Practice-Initiated Quality Improvement for Depression: Results of a Randomized Controlled Trial," *Journal of the American Medical Association* 286, no. 11 (September 19, 2001): 1325–1330.

30. Kessler et al., "The Epidemiology of Major Depressive Disorder" (see note 16, chapter 2), 3095–3105.

31. Considering the extensiveness of SSRI use, it is remarkable how little we know about their effectiveness in treating persons with acute minor depression. A recent randomized study of 162 patients treated with fluoxetine or placebo over twelve weeks showed statistically significant improvement over a number of measures, but the differences were modest in practical clinical terms. See Lewis L. Judd, Mark Hyman Rapaport, Kimberly A. Yonkers, et al., "Randomized, Placebo-Controlled

Trial of Fluoxetine for Acute Treatment of Minor Depressive Disorder," *American Journal of Psychiatry* 161, no. 10 (October 2004): 1864–1871.

32. Comorbid mental illness contributes significantly to role impairments associated with such disorders as arthritis, hypertension, asthma, and ulcers. See Ronald C. Kessler, Johan Ormel, Olga Demler, et al., "Comorbid Mental Disorders Account for the Role Impairment of Commonly Occurring Chronic Physical Disorders: Results from the National Comorbidity Survey," *Journal of Occupational and Environmental Medicine* 45, no. 12 (December 2003): 1257–1266.

33. David Mechanic, "Approaches for Coordinating Primary and Specialty Care for Persons with Mental Illness," *General Hospital Psychiatry* 19, no. 6 (November 1997): 395–402.

34. Mechanic, *Mental Health and Social Policy*.

35. New Freedom Commission on Mental Health, *Achieving the Promise: Transforming Mental Health Care in America*, final report, DHHS pub. no. SMA-03-3832 (Rockville, MD: U.S. Government Printing Office, 2003).

36. Linda A. Teplin, Gary M. McClelland, Karen M. Abram, et al., "Crime Victimization in Adults with Severe Mental Illness," *Archives of General Psychiatry* 62, no. 8 (August 2005): 911–921.

37. Catherine D. DeAngelis, Jeffrey M. Drazen, Frank A. Frizelle, et al., "Is This Clinical Trial Fully Registered?—A Statement From the International Committee of Medical Journal Editors," *New England Journal of Medicine* 352, no. 23 (June 9, 2005): 2436–2438.

38. Wang et al., "Twelve-Month Use of Mental Health Services in the United States," 629–640.

Chapter 5 — The Activated Patient and the Doctors' Dilemma

1. John Abramson, *Overdosed America: The Broken Promise of American Medicine* (New York: Harper Collins, 2004), xii. The book, an account of a doctor seeking to practice in a thoughtful evidence-based way, offers a variety of anecdotes of some of the difficulties in dealing with determined patients insisting on a medication they learned about through DTC advertising.

2. Talcott Parsons, *The Social System* (New York: Free Press, 1961).

3. Rosemary A. Stevens, "Medical Specialization as American Health Policy Interweaving Public and Private Roles," in *History and Health Policy in the United States*, ed. Rosemary A. Stevens, Charles E. Rosenberg, and Lawton R. Burns (New Brunswick, N.J.: Rutgers University Press, 2006); also see the updated edition of Rosemary A. Steven's classic *American Medicine and the Public Interest* (Berkeley: University of California Press, 1998).

4. Stevens, "Medical Specialization."

5. Dale A. Newton and Martha S. Grayson, "Trends in Career Choice by U.S. Medical School Graduates," *Journal of the American Medical Association* 290, no. 9 (September 3, 2003): 1179–1182.

6. Christine Wiebe, "Doctor Pay Surveys Reveal Growing Gaps," *Medscape Business of Medicine* 6, no. 1 (2005). Available online: www.medscape.com/viewarticle/501716.

7. Barbara Starfield, *Primary Care: Balancing Health Needs, Services, and Technology* (New York: Oxford University Press, 1998).

8. James Macinko, Barbara Starfield, and Leiyu Shi, "The Contribution of Primary Care Systems to Health Outcomes within Organization for Economic Cooperation and Development (OECD) Countries, 1970–1998," *Health Services Research* 38, no. 3 (June 2003): 831–865.

9. Marcia Angell, *The Truth About the Drug Companies: How They Deceive Us and What to Do About It* (New York: Random House, 2004), 121.

10. Ibid., 122.

11. Ibid., 124.

12. Jerry Avorn, *Powerful Medicines: The Benefits, Risks, and Costs of Prescription Drugs* (New York: Alfred A. Knopf, 2004).

13. Kassirer, *On the Take* (see note 31, chapter 1).

14. Many excellent books have been published on the pharmaceutical industry. I especially recommend Avorn, *Powerful Medicines*.

15. Rebecca Voelker, "Easy-To-Use Drug Reports Help Patients and Physicians Weigh Costs, Benefits," *Journal of the American Medical Association* 294, no. 2 (July 13, 2005): 165–166.

16. Joel S. Weissman, David Blumenthal, Alvin J. Silk, et al., "Physicians Report on Patient Encounters Involving Direct-to-Consumer Advertising," *Health Affairs Web Exclusive*, April 28, 2004. Available online: http://content.healthaffairs.org.

17. Abramson, *Overdosed America*.

18. David Mechanic, Donna D. McAlpine, and Marsha Rosenthal, "Are Patients' Office Visits with Physicians Getting Shorter?" *New England Journal of Medicine* 344, no 3 (January 18, 2001): 198–204.

19. David Mechanic, "Physician Discontent: Challenges and Opportunities," *Journal of the American Medical Association* 290, no. 7 (August 20, 2003): 941–946.

20. Kimberly S. H. Yarnall, Kathryn I. Pollak, Truls Østbye, et al., "Primary Care: Is There Enough Time for Prevention?" *American Journal of Public Health* 93, no. 4 (April 2003): 635–641.

21. Elizabeth A. McGlynn, Steven M. Asch, John Adams, et al., "The Quality of Health Care Delivered to Adults in the United States," *New England Journal of Medicine* 348, no. 26 (June 26, 2003): 2635–2645.

22. Robert Cunningham, "Professionalism Reconsidered: Physician Payment in a Small-Practice Environment," *Health Affairs* 23, no. 6 (November/December 2004): 36–47.

23. Sherrie H. Kaplan, Barbara Gandek, Sheldon Greenfield, et al., "Patient and Visit Characteristics Related to Physicians' Participatory Decision-Making Style: Results from the Medical Outcomes Study," *Medical Care* 33, no. 12 (December 1995): 1176–1187; for a more general review, see Debra L. Roter and Judith A. Hall, *Doctors Talking with Patients/Patients Talking with Doctors: Improving Communication in Medical Visits* (Westport, Conn.: Auburn House, 1992).

24. Researchers at the Center for the Evaluative Clinical Sciences at Dartmouth Medical School have done much work on this issue. For a summary of work on patient decision aids, see Annette M. O'Connor, Hilary A. Llewellyn-Thomas, and Ann Barry Flood, "Modifying Unwarranted Variations in Health Care: Shared Decision Making Using Patient Decision Aids," *Health Affairs Web Exclusive*, October 7, 2004. Available online: http://content.healthaffairs.org.

25. George C. Halvorson and George J. Isham, *Epidemic of Care: A Call for Safer, Better and More Accountable Health Care* (San Francisco: Jossey-Bass, 2003).

26. Jonathan B. Perlin, Robert M. Kolodner, and Robert H. Roswell, "The Veterans Health Administration: Quality, Value, Accountability, and Information as Transforming Strategies for Patient-Centered Care," *American Journal of Managed Care* 10, no. 11, part 2 (November 2004): 828–836.

27. Alain C. Enthoven, Laura A. Tollen, and William L. Roper, eds., *Toward a 21st Cen-

tury Health System: The Contributions and Promise of Prepaid Group Practice (San Francisco: Jossey-Bass, 2004).

28. Diane R. Rittenhouse, Kevin Grumbach, Edward H. O'Neil, et al., "Physician Organization and Care Management in California: From Cottage to Kaiser," *Health Affairs* 23, no. 6 (November/December 2004): 51–62.

29. Bruce Fireman, Joan Bartlett, and Joe Selby, "Can Disease Management Reduce Health Care Costs by Improving Quality?" *Health Affairs* 23, no. 6 (November/December 2004): 63–75.

30. See Avorn, *Powerful Medicines*, particularly 314–338.

31. As one might expect, an endeavor like NICE gets mixed reviews. See Michael D. Rawlins, "NICE Work-Providing Guidance to the British National Health Service," *New England Journal of Medicine* 351, no. 14 (September 30, 2004): 1383–1385; Also see Trevor A. Sheldon, Nicky Cullum, Diane Dawson, et al., "What's the Evidence that NICE Guidance Has Been Implemented? Results from a National Evaluation Using Time Series Analysis, Audit of Patients' Notes and Interviews," *British Medical Journal* 329, no. 7473 (October 30, 2004): 999–1003.

32. For an introduction to the Cochrane Collaboration, go to www.cochrane.org .

33. See Avorn, *Powerful Medicines*; Angell, *The Truth About the Drug Companies*; Abramson, *Overdosed America*; also see Merrill Goozner, *The $800 Million Pill: The Truth Behind the Cost of New Drugs* (Berkeley: University of California Press, 2004).

34. Frank Davidoff, Catherine D. DeAngelis, Jeffrey M. Drazen, et al, "Sponsorship, Authorship, and Accountability," *New England Journal of Medicine* 345, no. 11 (September 13, 2001): 825–826.

35. Angell, *The Truth About the Drug Companies*, xviii.

36. Kassirer, *On the Take*.

Chapter 6 — The Neglect of Long-Term Care

1. Jerald Winakur, "What Are We Going to Do with Dad?" *Health Affairs* 24, no. 4 (July/August 2005): 1064–1072.

2. For a very thoughtful picture of the challenges of caring for patients with increasing dementia and the stresses placed on family members and caretakers, see Muriel R. Gillick, *Tangled Minds: Understanding Alzheimer's Disease and Other Dementias* (New York: Dutton, 1998).

3. This is not to suggest that there have not been thoughtful and important policy proposals. One of my favorite analyses is Robert M. Ball and Thomas N. Bethell, *Because We're All in This Together: The Case for a National Long Term Care Insurance Policy* (Washington, D.C.: Families USA Foundation, 1989).

4. For an overall evaluation of the program, and future potential, see Nelda McCall, ed., *Who Will Pay for Long-Term Care? Insights from the Partnership Programs* (Chicago: Health Administration Press, 2001).

5. Ellen O'Brien and Risa Elias, *Medicaid and Long-Term Care* (Kaiser Commission on Medicaid and the Uninsured, Washington, D.C.: Henry J. Kaiser Family Foundation, May 2004). This informative report includes much useful data on the Medicaid program, and I draw on it throughout the chapter.

6. Ibid.

7. See Rosalie A. Kane, Richard L. Kane, and Richard C. Ladd, *The Heart of Long-Term Care* (New York: Oxford University Press, 1998).

8. Wendy Fox-Grage, Donna Folkemer, and Jordan Lewis, "The States' Response to the *Olmstead* Decision: How Are States Complying?" National Conference of State Leg-

islatures. Available online: www.ncsl.org; also see Sara Rosenbaum, "The Olmstead Decision: Implications for State Health Policy," *Health Affairs* 19, no. 5 (September/October 2000): 228–232.

9. Peter Kemper, Robert Applebaum, and Mary Harrigan, "Community Care Demonstrations: What Have We Learned?" *Health Care Financing Review* 8, no. 4 (Summer 1987): 87–100; Jon B. Christianson, The Evaluation of the National Long-Term Caregiving Demonstration 6. The Effect of Channeling on Informal Care," *Health Services Research* 23, no. 1 (April 1988): 99–117.

10. Joshua M. Wiener and Jason Skaggs, *Current Approaches to Integrating Acute and Long-Term Care Financing and Services*, publication no. 9516 (Washington, D.C.: American Association of Retired Persons, 1995).

11. Diane L. Gross, Helena Temkin-Greener, Stephen Kunitz, et al., "The Growing Pains of Integrated Health Care for the Elderly: Lessons from the Expansion of PACE," *Milbank Quarterly* 82, no. 2 (June 2004): 257–282.

12. Ibid.

13. Charlene Harrington and Robert J. Newcomer, "Social Health Maintenance Organizations," *Generations* 14, no. 2 (Spring 1990): 49–54; Charlene Harrington and Robert J. Newcomer, "Social Health Maintenance Organizations' Service Use and Costs, 1985–1989," *Health-Care Financing Review* 12, no. 3 (Spring 1991): 37–52.

14. David Mechanic, "Policy Challenges in Improving Mental Health Services: Some Lessons From the Past," *Psychiatric Services* 54, no. 9 (September 2003): 1227–1232.

15. Jerry L. Mashaw and Virginia P. Reno, eds., *Balancing Security and Opportunity: The Challenge of Disability Income Policy* (Washington, D.C.: National Academy of Social Insurance, 1996). See chapter 6, "Vocational Rehabilitation and Return to Work Services: Fostering Innovation," 101–119.

16. See, for example, Judith H. Hibbard, Paul Slovic, Ellen Peters, et al., "Is the Informed-Choice Policy Approach Appropriate for Medicare Beneficiaries?" *Health Affairs* 20, no. 3 (May/June 2001): 199–203.

17. See, for example, Christine E. Bishop, "Where Are the Missing Elders? The Decline in Nursing Home Use, 1985 and 1995," *Health Affairs* 18, no. 4 (July/August 1999): 146–155.

18. Committee on Nursing Home Regulation, Institute of Medicine, *Improving the Quality of Care in Nursing Homes* (Washington, D.C.: National Academies Press, 1986).

19. O'Brien and Elias, *Medicaid and Long-Term Care.*

20. Joshua M. Weiner and David G. Stevenson, *Repeal of the Boren Amendment: Implications for Quality of Care in Nursing Homes*, December 1, 1998. Available online: www.urban.org.

21. Vincent Mor, Jacqueline Zinn, Joseph Angelelli, et al., "Driven to Tiers: Socioeconomic and Racial Disparities in the Quality of Nursing Home Care," *Milbank Quarterly* 82, no. 2 (June 2004): 227–256.

22. Ibid.

23. Those who wish to learn more about the Institute can visit its Web site at www.hartfordign.org.

24. The Eden Alternative, available online: www.edenalt.com.

25. See Kane et al., *The Heart of Long-Term Care*, 173–174.

26. To learn more about this effort, see http://thegreenhouseproject.com.

27. http://thegreenhouseproject.com.

28. Robyn I. Stone, Susan C. Reinhard, Barbara Bowers, et al., *Evaluation of the Well-spring Model for Improving Nursing Home Quality* (New York: Commonwealth Fund, August 2002).

Chapter 7 — The Quest for Quality

1. David L. Sackett, William M. C. Rosenberg, J. A. Muir Gray, et al., "Evidence-Based Medicine: What It Is and What It Isn't," *British Medical Journal* 312, no. 7023 (January 13, 1996): 71–72.
2. Kohn et al., *To Err Is Human* (see note 14, introduction).
3. Leape, "Preventing Medical Errors" (see note 15, introduction).
4. Mark A. Schuster, Elizabeth A. McGlynn, and Robert H. Brook, "How Good Is the Quality of Health Care in the United States?" *Milbank Quarterly* 76, no. 4 (December 1998): 517–563.
5. Elizabeth A. McGlynn, Steven M. Asch, John Adams, et al., "The Quality of Health Care Delivered to Adults in the United States," *New England Journal of Medicine* 348, no. 26 (June 26, 2003): 2635–2645.
6. Ibid., 2644.
7. Milton I. Roemer, "Bed Supply and Hospital Utilization: A Natural Experiment," *Hospitals, The Journal of the American Hospital Association* 35, no. 21 (November 1, 1961): 36–42.
8. John P. Bunker, "Surgical Manpower: A Comparison of Operations and Surgeons in the United States and in England and Wales," *New England Journal of Medicine* 282, no. 3 (January 15, 1970): 135–144.
9. John Wennberg and Alan Gittelsohn, "Small Area Variations in Health Care Delivery," *Science* 182, no. 4117 (December 14, 1973): 1102–1108.
10. Fitzhugh Mullan, "Wrestling with Variation: An Interview with Jack Wennberg," *Health Affairs Web Exclusive*, October 7, 2004. Available online: http://content.healthaffairs.org.
11. The health policy journal *Health Affairs* has devoted two special issues to practice variations, the first in the summer of 1984 and more recently in 2004.
12. See especially Elliott S. Fisher, David E. Wennberg, Therese A. Stukel, et al., "Variations in the Longitudinal Efficiency of Academic Medical Centers," *Health Affairs Web Exclusive*, October 7, 2004. Available online: http://content.healthaffairs.org.
13. Mary E. Tinetti, Sidney T. Bogardus, Jr., and Joseph V. Agostini, "Potential Pitfalls of Disease-Specific Guidelines for Patients with Multiple Conditions," *New England Journal of Medicine* 351, no. 27 (December 30, 2004): 2870–2874.
14. Abramson, *Overdosed America* (see note 1, chapter 5), 143.
15. Michael E. Mendelsohn and Richard H. Karas, "Molecular and Cellular Basis of Cardiovascular Gender Differences," *Science* 308, no. 5728 (June 10, 2005): 1583–1587.
16. Jocelyn Kaiser, "Gender in the Pharmacy: Does it Matter?" *Science* 308, no. 5728 (June 10, 2005): 1572–1574.
17. Paul M. Ridker, Nancy R. Cook, I-Min Lee, et al., "A Randomized Trial of Low-Dose Aspirin in the Primary Prevention of Cardiovascular Disease in Women," *New England Journal of Medicine* 352, no. 13 (March 31, 2005): 1293–1304.
18. Anne L. Taylor, Susan Ziesche, Clyde Yancy, et al., "Combination of Isosorbide Dinitrate and Hydralazine in Blacks with Heart Failure," *New England Journal of Medicine* 351, no. 20 (November 11, 2004): 2049–2057.
19. M. Gregg Bloche, "Race-Based Therapeutics," *New England Journal of Medicine* 351, no. 20 (November 11, 2004): 2035–2037.

20. Patrick J. O'Connor, "Adding Value to Evidence-Based Clinical Guidelines," *Journal of the American Medical Association* 294, no. 6 (August 10, 2005): 741–743.

21. Cynthia M. Boyd, Jonathan Darer, Chad Boult, et al., "Clinical Practice Guidelines and Quality of Care for Older Patients with Multiple Comorbid Diseases: Implications for Pay for Performance," *Journal of the American Medical Association* 294, no. 6 (August 10, 2005): 716–724.

22. Allan Korn, "Professionalism Reconsidered: Physician Payment From A Health Plan Perspective," *Health Affairs* 23, no. 6 (November/December 2004): 48–50.

23. For a thoughtful debate on these issues, see Robert A. Berenson, "Paying for Quality and Doing It Right," *Washington and Lee Law Review* 60, no. 4 (Fall 2003): 1315–1344, and Bruce C. Vladeck, "If Paying for Quality Is Such a Bad Idea, Why Is Everyone for It?" *Washington and Lee Law Review* 60, no. 4 (Fall 2003): 1345–1372.

24. UK Department of Health, *Investing in General Practice: The New GMS Contract* (London: DOH, 2003); see also Peter C. Smith and Nick York, "Quality Incentives: The Case of UK General Practitioners," *Health Affairs* 23, no. 3 (May/June 2004): 112–118.

25. Smith and York, "Quality Incentives," 114.

26. Morris Weinberger, ed., "Consumer Assessment of Health Plans Study (CAHPS™), *Medical Care* 37, no. 3, Supplement (March 1999).

27. Major influences include the Institute of Medicine of the National Academy of Sciences (Institute of Medicine, *Crossing the Quality Chasm: A New Health System for the 21st Century* [Washington, D.C.: National Academies Press, 2001]) and National Committee for Quality Assurance (Eric C. Schneider, Virginia Riehl, Sonja Courte-Wienecke, et al., "Enhancing Performance Measurement: NCQA's Road Map for a Health Information Framework," *Journal of the American Medical Association* 282, no. 12 [September 22, 1999]: 1184–1190).

28. Mark R. Chassin, "Quality of Health Care. Part 3: Improving the Quality of Care," *New England Journal of Medicine* 335, no. 14 (October 3, 1996): 1060–1063.

29. Berenson, "Paying for Quality," 1315–1344, and Vladeck, "If Paying for Quality Is Such a Bad Idea?" 1345–1372.

30. Henry J. Kaiser Family Foundation/Agency for Healthcare Research and Quality. *National Survey on Americans as Health Care Consumers: An Update on the Role of Quality Information.* Conducted July 31–October 9, 2000.

31. Ibid.

32. Lawrence K. Altman, "Clinton Surgery Puts Attention on Death Rate," *New York Times*, September 6, 2004, late edition, final, section A, page 1, column 1.

33. Barry Schwartz, Andrew Ward, John Monterosso, et al., "Maximizing Versus Satisficing: Happiness Is a Matter of Choice," *Journal of Personality and Social Psychology* 83, no. 5 (November 2002): 1178–1197. Also see Barry Schwartz, *The Paradox of Choice: Why More Is Less* (New York: Ecco, 2004).

34. David Mechanic, "Physician Discontent: Challenges and Opportunities," *Journal of the American Medical Association* 290, no. 7 (August 20, 2003): 941–946.

35. David Mechanic and William Parson, "Shortcuts Are Not Necessarily Bad," *Journal of Medical Education* 50, no. 6 (June 1975): 638–639.

36. Rosemary A. Stevens, "Specialization, Specialty Organizations, and the Quality of Health Care," in Mechanic et al., *Policy Challenges* (see note 15, introduction), 206–220.

Chapter 8 — Setting Fair Limits

1. Robert Salladay, "Gov. Says No to Viagra for Sex Offenders," *Los Angeles Times*, May 27, 2005. Available online: http://www.latimes.com.

2. Todd Zwillich, "House Vote Bars Impotence Drugs From Medicare," WebMDHealth, June 24, 2005. Available online: http://my.webmd.com.

3. Tom Curry, "Worry Builds in Congress Over Massive Cost of New Drug Entitlement." Available online: http://msnbc.com.

4. Rudolf Klein and Heidrun Sturm, "Viagra: A Success Story for Rationing?" *Health Affairs* 21, no. 6 (November/December 2002): 177–187.

5. Ibid., 184.

6. Rudolf Klein, Patricia Day, and Sharon Redmayne, *Managing Scarcity: Priority Setting and Rationing in the National Health Service* (Philadelphia: Open University Press, 1996).

7. Ibid., 68.

8. See, for example, Kenneth I. Howard, Thomas A. Cornille, John S. Lyons, et al., "Patterns of Mental Health Service Utilization," *Archives of General Psychiatry* 53, no. 8 (August 1996): 696–703.

9. For example, comparisons with Canada, using similar methodology, show that services are disproportionately used by those with lesser need in the United States. See Ronald C. Kessler, Richard G. Frank, Mark Edlund, et al., "Differences in the Use of Psychiatric Outpatient Services between the United States and Ontario," *New England Journal of Medicine* 336, no. 8 (February 20, 1997): 551–557.

10. David Mechanic, "Muddling Through Elegantly: Finding the Proper Balance in Rationing," *Health Affairs* 16, no. 5 (September/October 1997): 83–92.

11. For an interesting exposition on cultural differences in treatment values and preferences, see Lynn Payer, *Medicine and Culture: Varieties of Treatment in the United States, England, West Germany, and France* (New York: Henry Holt, 1988). Payer notes that after World War II, the Sécurité Sociale decided to reimburse the costs of spa treatment in France and that in 1984 half a million people took such treatments, with 95 percent partially reimbursed by health insurance (71–72). She also notes that medical use of spas is even more widespread in Germany (96).

12. For a thoughtful and comprehensive account of these arrangements, see Rudolf Klein, *The New Politics of the National Health Service*, 3rd ed. (London: Longman, 1995).

13. For an examination of rationing of dialysis in the National Health Service, see Henry J. Aaron and William B. Schwartz, *The Painful Prescription: Rationing Hospital Care* (Washington, D.C.: The Brookings Institution, 1984).

14. For a discussion of some of the advantages of implicit rationing, see David Mechanic, "Dilemmas in Rationing Health Care Services: The Case for Implicit Rationing," *British Medical Journal* 310, no. 6995 (24 June 1995): 1655–1659.

15. For example, see Thomas Halper, *The Misfortunes of Others: End-Stage Renal Disease in the United Kingdom* (Cambridge, UK: Cambridge University Press, 1989).

16. See, for example, Trevor A. Sheldon and Alan Maynard, "Is Rationing Inevitable?" in *Rationing in Action*, ed. Richard Smith (London: BMJ Publishing Group, 1993), 3–14.

17. Mechanic, "The Rise and Fall of Managed Care" (see note 9, introduction).

18. Lawrence D. Brown, "The National Politics of Oregon's Rationing Plan," *Health Affairs* 10, no. 2 (Summer 1991): 28–51; U.S. Congress Office of Technology Assess-

ment, *Evaluation of the Oregon Medicaid Proposal, OTA-H-531* (Washington, D.C.: U.S. Government Printing Office, May 1992).

19. David C. Hadorn, "Setting Health Care Priorities in Oregon: Cost-Effectiveness Meets the Rule of Rescue," *Journal of the American Medical Association* 265, no. 17 (May 1, 1991): 2218–2225.

20. Lawrence Jacobs, Theodore Marmor, and Jonathan Oberlander, "The Oregon Health Plan and the Political Paradox of Rationing: What Advocates and Critics Have Claimed and What Oregon Did," *Journal of Health Politics, Policy and Law* 24, no. 1 (February 1999): 161–180.

21. Howard M. Leichter, "Oregon's Bold Experiment: Whatever Happened to Rationing?" *Journal of Health Politics, Policy and Law* 24, no. 1 (February 1999): 147–160.

22. Jacobs et al., "The Oregon Health Plan," 161–180.

23. Guido Calabresi and Philip Bobbitt, *Tragic Choices* (New York: W. W. Norton, 1978).

24. Jon Elster, *Local Justice: How Institutions Allocate Scarce Goods and Necessary Burdens* (New York: Russell Sage Foundation, 1992).

25. James Walkup, Usha Sambamoorthi, and Stephen Crystal, "Incidence and Consistency of Antiretroviral Use Among HIV-Infected Medicaid Beneficiaries with Schizophrenia," *Journal of Clinical Psychiatry* 62, no. 3 (March 2001): 174–178.

26. See Klein et al., *Managing Scarcity*, 77–81, and Vikki A. Entwistle, Ian S. Watt, Richard Bradbury, et al., "Media Coverage of the Child B. Case," *British Medical Journal* 312, no. 7046 (June 22, 1996): 1587–1591.

27. Law Report, *Times* (London), March 15, 1995, p. 23.

28. A 1996 survey of twelve large health plans by the General Accounting Office found that nine indicated that threat of litigation was a major factor in decisions to cover chemotherapy plus autologous bone marrow transplant. See Michelle M. Mello and Troyen A. Brennan, "The Controversy Over High-Dose Chemotherapy with Autologous Bone Marrow Transplant for Breast Cancer," *Health Affairs* 20, no. 5 (September/October 2001): 101–117.

29. Sharon Redmayne, Rudolf Klein, and Patricia Day, *Sharing Our Resources: Purchasing and Priority Setting in the National Health Service*, research paper no. 11 (Birmingham, UK: National Association of Health Authorities and Trusts, 1993); see also Klein and Sturm, "Viagra," 177–187.

30. Norman Daniels and James E. Sabin, *Setting Limits Fairly: Can We Learn to Share Medical Resources?* (New York: Oxford University Press, 2002).

31. Norman Daniels, "Accountability for Reasonable Limits to Care: Can We Meet the Challenges?" in Mechanic et al., *Policy Challenges* (see note 15, introduction), 238–248.

Chapter 9 — Restoring Trust in the Health System

1. The survey was conducted by National Opinion Research Center, University of Chicago, February 6–June 26, 2002, and based on personal interviews with a national adult sample of 2,765. Data provided by the Roper Center for Public Opinion Research, University of Connecticut. Available online: www.ropercenter.uconn.edu.

2. Ronald Inglehart, "Postmateralist Values and the Erosion of Institutional Authority," in *Why People Don't Trust Government*, ed. Joseph S. Nye, Jr., Philip D. Zelikow, and David C. King (Cambridge: Harvard University Press, 1997), 217–236.

3. Carol Cruzan Morton, "Research Briefs: Initiative Looks for Ways to Build Trust,"

Focus: News From Harvard Medical, Dental and Public Health Schools, January 24, 2003. Available online: http://focus.hms.harvard.edu. Physicians have had high prestige for some time. For comparable assessment of occupations, see Robert W. Hodge, Paul M. Siegel, Peter H. Rossi, "Occupational Prestige in the United States, 1925–63," *American Journal of Sociology* 70, no. 3 (November 1964): 286–302.

4. Starr, *The Social Transformation of American Medicine* (see note 20, chapter 1).
5. Morton, "Research Briefs."
6. Gary Orren, "Fall From Grace: The Public's Loss of Faith in Government," in Nye et al., *Why People Don't Trust Government*, 81.
7. Ibid.
8. Morton, "Research Briefs."
9. Suzanne L. Parker and Glenn R. Parker, "Why Do We Trust Our Congressman?" *Journal of Politics* 55, no. 2 (May 1993): 442–453.
10. Lawrence R. Jacobs and Robert Y. Shapiro, *Politicians Don't Pander* (Chicago: University of Chicago Press, 2000), 237.
11. Seymour M. Lipset, "Malaise and Resiliency in America," *Journal of Democracy* 6, no. 3 (July 1995): 4–18.
12. Robert D. Putnam, *Bowling Alone: The Collapse and Revival of American Community* (New York: Simon and Schuster, 2000).
13. Marsha Rosenthal, "Older Patients' Trust and Disrupted Trust in Doctors and Health Plans: Determinants and Implications" (Ph.D. diss., Rutgers University, 2004).
14. David Mechanic and Sharon Meyer, "Concepts of Trust Among Patients with Serious Illness," *Social Science and Medicine* 51, no. 5 (September 1, 2000): 657–668.
15. Julie Schmittdiel, Joe V. Selby, Kevin Grumbach, et al., "Choice of a Personal Physician and Patient Satisfaction in a Health Maintenance Organization," *Journal of the American Medical Association* 278, no. 19 (November 19, 1997): 1596–1599.
16. Mechanic and Meyer, "Concepts of Trust," 657–668.
17. Mechanic, "The Functions and Limitations of Trust in the Provision of Medical Care" (see note 38, chapter 1).
18. Mechanic and Meyer, "Concepts of Trust," 657–668.
19. Debra L. Roter and Judith A. Hall, *Doctors Talking with Patients/Patients Talking with Doctors* (Westport, Conn.: Auburn House, 1992).
20. Mechanic and Meyer, "Concepts of Trust," 657–668.
21. In recent years there has been increasingly serious conflicts of interests in medicine. See Kassirer, *On the Take* (see note 31, chapter 1).
22. For two important statements on this issue, see Institute of Medicine, Committee on Quality of Health Care in America, *Crossing the Quality Chasm* (see note 27, chapter 7), and Kohn et al., *To Err Is Human* (see note 14, introduction).
23. David Mechanic and Mark Schlesinger, "The Impact of Managed Care on Patients' Trust in Medical Care and Their Physicians," *Journal of the American Medical Association* 275, no. 21 (June 5, 1996): 1693–1697.
24. Susan P. Shapiro, "The Social Control of Impersonal Trust," *American Journal of Sociology* 93 (November 1987): 623–658.
25. Marc A. Rodwin, *Medicine, Money and Morals: Physicians' Conflicts of Interest* (New York: Oxford University Press, 1993).
26. For a classic statement on this issue, see Stewart Macaulay, "Non-Contractual Relations in Business," *American Sociological Review* 28, no. 1 (February 1963): 55–67, and Stewart Macaulay, *Law and the Balance of Power: The Automobile Manufacturers and Their Dealers* (New York: Russell Sage Foundation, 1966).

27. Inglehart, "Postmateralist Values and the Erosion of Institutional Authority," 217–236.

28. The phrase comes from David Halberstam's book, *The Best and the Brightest* (New York: Random House, 1972), which reviews the Vietnam War and how it was represented to the public.

29. See Kassirer, *On the Take*; also see Abramson, *Overdosed America* (see note 1, chapter 5), and Angell, *The Truth About the Drug Companies* (see note 9, chapter 5).

30. Derek C. Bok, *Universities in the Marketplace: The Commercialization of Higher Education* (Princeton, N.J.: Princeton University Press, 2003); also see Daniel S. Greenberg, *Science, Money and Politics: Political Triumph and Ethical Erosion* (Chicago: University of Chicago Press, 2001).

31. Arnold S. Relman, "The Health of Nations: Medicine and the Free Market," *New Republic* 232, no. 8 (March 7, 2005): 23–30.

32. Rosemary A. Stevens, "Specialization, Specialty Organizations, and the Quality of Health Care," in Mechanic et al., *Policy Challenges* (see note 15, introduction), 206–220.

33. James C. Robinson, "Entrepreneurial Challenges to Integrated Health Care," in Mechanic et al., *Policy Challenges* (see note 15, introduction), 53–67.

34. See, for example, Barron H. Lerner, *The Breast Cancer Wars: Hope, Fear, and the Pursuit of a Cure in Twentieth-Century America* (New York: Oxford University Press, 2001).

35. George C. Halvorson and George J. Isham, *Epidemic of Care: A Call for Safer, Better, and More Accountable Health Care* (San Francisco: Jossey-Bass, 2003).

36. David Mechanic and Marsha Rosenthal, "Responses of HMO Medical Directors to Trust Building in Managed Care," *Milbank Quarterly* 77, no. 3 (September 1999): 283–303.

37. Mark Schlesinger, Bradford H. Gray, and Michael Gusmano, "A Broader Vision for Managed Care, Part 3: The Scope and Determinants of Community Benefits," *Health Affairs* 23, no. 3 (May/June 2004): 210–221.

38. Medical Professionalism Project, "Medical Professionalism in the New Millennium: A Physicians' Charter," *The Lancet* 359, no. 9305 (February 9, 2002): 520–522.

39. Stevens, "Specialization, Specialty Organizations, and the Quality of Health Care, " 218.

Part III — The Fork in the Road

1. Kaiser Health Poll Report, "The Public's Assessment of the State of U.S. Health Care." Available online: www.kff.org.

2. Kaiser Health Poll Report, "Most Important Problem for Government to Address—Trends." Available online: www.kff.org.

3. Theda Skocpol, *Boomerang: Health Care Reform and the Turn Against Government* (New York: W. W. Norton, 1997), 109.

Chapter 10 — The Challenge of Change

1. There is much data available on insurance coverage. Both the Henry J. Kaiser Family Foundation (www.kff.org) and the Commonwealth Fund (www.cmwf.org) provide abundant information through their Web sites.

2. Reporting on a study by the Urban Institute and the University of Minnesota's State Health Access Data Assistance Center, "Number of Uninsured Children Down, But Too Many Still Not in Public Programs, Report Says." Available online: http://www.cmwf.org.

3. Lynn M. Olson, Suk-fong S. Tang, and Paul W. Newacheck, "Children in the United States with Discontinuous Health Insurance Coverage," *New England Journal of Medicine* 353, no. 4 (July 28, 2005): 382–391.

4. In 2003, 70 percent of uninsured persons came from families in which there was a full-time worker, and only one-fifth of the uninsured were in families unconnected to the work force. See Kaiser Commission on Medicaid and the Uninsured, *The Uninsured: A Primer* (Washington, D.C.: Kaiser Family Foundation, November 2004).

5. Rainu Kaushal, David Blumenthal, Eric G. Poon, et al., "The Costs of a National Health Information Network," *Annals of Internal Medicine* 143, no. 3 (August 2, 2005): 165–173.

6. These experiences are reviewed in Deyo and Patrick, *Hope or Hype* (see note 17, chapter 1).

7. Edward A. Stadtmauer, Anne O'Neill, Lori J. Goldstein, et al., "Conventional-Dose Chemotherapy Compared with High-Dose Chemotherapy Plus Autologous Hematopoietic Stem-Cell Transplantation for Metastatic Breast Cancer," *New England Journal of Medicine* 342, no. 15 (April 13, 2000): 1069–1076.

8. Robert E. Mechanic, *Disease Management: A Promising Approach for Health Care Purchasers*, executive brief (Washington, D.C.: National Health Care Purchasing Institute, May 2002).

9. The RWJF program, Improving Chronic Illness Care, presents information about the program and about chronic disease on its Web site, www.improvingchroniccare.org.

10. Lawrence P. Casalino, "Disease Management and the Organization of Physician Practice," *Journal of the American Medical Association* 293, no. 4 (January 26, 2005): 485–488.

11. Ibid.

12. John Kralewski and Bryan E. Dowd, "Drug Errors in Medical Practices: It's Dangerous out There," research brief 12, no. 4 (University of Minnesota, Division of Health Services Research and Policy, July 2005).

13. As noted earlier, a large number of recently published books seek to bring these issues to broad public attention. Among these are Avorn, *Powerful Medicines* (see note 12, chapter 5); Abramson, *Overdosed America* (see note 1, chapter 5); Angell, *The Truth About Drug Companies* (see note 9, chapter 5); and Deyo and Patrick, *Hope or Hype*.

14. Phil B. Fontanarosa, Drummond Rennie, and Catherine D. DeAngelis, "Postmarketing Surveillance—Lack of Vigilance, Lack of Trust," *Journal of the American Medical Association* 292, no. 21 (December 1, 2004): 2647–2650.

15. Eric J. Topol, "Failing the Public Health—Rofecoxib, Merck, and the FDA," *New England Journal of Medicine* 351, no. 17 (October 21, 2004): 1707–1709.

16. Kassirer, *On the Take* (see note 31, chapter 1).

17. "US. Doctors Rebuff Drug Watchdog Group," *British Medical Journal* 330, no. 7496 (April 16, 2005): 862.

18. Steffie Woolhandler, Terry Campbell, and David U. Himmelstein, "Costs of Health Care Administration in the United States and Canada," *New England Journal of Medicine* 349, no. 8 (August 21, 2003): 768–775.

19. Ibid.

20. Kenneth E. Thorpe, "Inside the Black Box of Administrative Costs," *Health Affairs* 11, no. 2 (Summer 1992): 41–55.

21. Skocpol, *Boomerang* (see note 3, part 3).

22. For a forceful statement of this issue, see Deyo and Patrick, *Hope or Hype*.

23. W. Grant Thompson, *The Placebo Effect and Health: Combining Science and Compassionate Care* (New York: Prometheus Books, 2005).

24. Michael J. Barry, Floyd J. Fowler Jr., Albert G. Mulley, Jr., et al., "Patient Reactions to a Program Designed to Facilitate Patient Participation in Treatment Decisions for Benign Prostatic Hyperplasia," *Medical Care* 33, no. 8 (August 1995): 771–782.

25. Annette M. Cormier O'Connor, Alaa Rostom, Jacqueline Tetroe, et al., "Effectiveness of Decision Aids for People Facing Health Treatment or Screening Decisions." Abstract: Cochrane Review. www.cochrane.org.

26. Paula M. Lantz, Nancy K. Janz, Angela Fagerlin, et al., "Satisfaction with Surgery Outcomes and the Decision Process in a Population-Based Sample of Women with Breast Cancer," *Health Services Research* 40, no. 3 (June 2005): 745–767.

Chapter 11 — Steps in Our Health Future

1. Arnold S. Relman, "The Health of Nations: Medicine and the Free Market," *The New Republic* 232, no. 8 (March 7, 2005): 23–30.

2. Gail R. Wilensky, "The Nation's Health Policy Agenda: Real—and Realistic—Opportunities for Progress." Available online: http://www.cmwf.org.

3. Brian Biles, Lauren Hersch Nicholas, and Barbara S. Cooper, *The Cost of Privatization: Extra Payments to Medicare Advantage Plans—2005 Update*, issue brief, publication no. 750 (New York: The Commonwealth Fund, December, 2004).

4. Henry J. Kaiser Family Foundation, publication no. 1066-08, *Fact Sheet: Medicare at a Glance* (Menlo Park, Calif.: April, 2005). Available online: www.kff.org.

5. Ibid.

6. Henry J. Kaiser Family Foundation, *Medicaid: An Overview of Spending on "Mandatory" vs. "Optional" Populations and Services*, issue paper (Washington, D.C.: Kaiser Commission on Medicaid and the Uninsured, June 2005).

7. Vernon K. Smith and Greg Moody, *Medicaid in 2005: Principles and Proposals for Reform* (Lansing, Mich.: Health Management Associates, February 2005).

8. Ibid.

9. National Governors Association, *Medicaid Reform: A Preliminary Report*. Available online: http://www.nga.org.

10. Linda H. Aiken, "Improving Quality through Nursing," in Mechanic et al., *Policy Challenges* (see note 15, introduction), 177–188.

Index

AARP, 15

ABMS (American Board of Medical Specialties), 86, 158

Abramson, John, 84, 119

accountability: "for reasonableness," 140; of physicians, 21, 108, 118, 129, 158; and social trust, 153. *See also* ethics (medical)

adolescents, 78

advanced directives, 10

advertising (marketing): amount of money spent by pharmaceutical companies on, 89–91, 96, 173; as an administrative cost, 175; creating demand for new technologies through, 24, 29, 90, 177; direct-to-consumer drug, 1–3, 12, 14, 25, 35, 77, 81, 84, 89–91, 93, 118, 130–31, 145, 171, 173, 174; drug trials oriented toward, 97–98; false or misleading, 2, 38, 98, 119, 155, 172, 174; against health care change, 159; of hospitals, 152; influence of, on individuals' behavior, 7, 8, 18, 50, 165. *See also* profits

Aetna, 15

affective psychoses, 72, 74

AFL-CIO, 15

African Americans, 7, 55, 60, 61–62, 119

Africans, 53, 61

age: and blood pressure, 53; and erectile dysfunction, 130; as factor in inequality of health care, 142; as factor in treatment plans, 118–19; health rationing by, 134; and homicide risk, 51; increasing, of American population, 8, 12, 23, 29, 51, 101; and pollution susceptibility, 56, 65; of underinsured persons, 23; of uninsured persons, 6. *See also* adolescents; children; elderly; infants; retirees

Agency for Healthcare Research and Quality (formerly Agency for Health Care Policy and Research), 19–20, 32–34, 120, 123

AIDS (HIV), 13, 63, 81, 89, 137, 156

air bags (in automobiles), 63

alcohol. *See* substance abuse

Aleve (drug). *See* naproxen

allocation (of health care). *See* rationing (of health care)

alternative and complementary medicine, 17, 68, 83, 177

Alzheimer's disease, 104. *See also* dementia

American Academy of Orthopaedic Surgeons, 20

American Board of Internal Medicine, 157

American Board of Medical Genetics, 88

American Board of Medical Specialties (ABMS), 86, 158

American Cancer Society, 15, 81

American College of Physicians (ACP), 157, 173–74

American Hospital Association, 15

American Medical Association, 15, 147

American Nursing Association, 15

American Psychiatric Association, 71. *See also* DSM-IV

American Public Health Association, 15

Americans with Disabilities Act, 103

Angell, Marcia, 89, 98

Anthem Blue Cross and Blue Shield, 15

antibiotics, 13

antidepressants, 77, 91. *See also* Fluoxetine (drug); SSRIs

antipsychotic drugs, 77

anxiety, 69, 78. *See also* panic disorder

appendectomies, 136

Asians, 55, 61, 105

aspirin, 42, 53

assisted-living facilities, 101, 103, 104–5, 112. *See also* long-term care

asthma, 34, 49, 199n32

atrial fibrillation, 116

autonomy: as health factor, 57–59; of physicians, 27–28, 127, 135, 140, 156, 164–65

avian flu, 13, 54

Aymara Indians, 41

back pain and surgery, 19–20

Balanced Budget Amendment (1997), 37, 105

Balint groups, 196n6

Becher, Elise, 21

Beecher, Henry, 44

benefits management, 175

Bergman, Abraham, 25

Bextra (drug), 91

BiDil (drug), 119

bipolar disease, 71, 72, 74

bird flu virus, 13, 54

blood lipid levels. *See* cholesterol (high)

blood pressure. *See* hypertension

Blue Cross, 15

bone marrow transplants, 137, 138–39, 167, 206n28

Boren Amendment, 108–9

breast cancer, 25, 89, 116, 156, 177–78; bone marrow transplants for, 139, 167, 206n28. *See also* mammography; radical mastectomies

Bunker, John, 117

burn units, 21

Bush, George W., 46, 131, 180; on mental health, 80–81, 106, 107; and privatization, 12, 107, 180–81

CAHPS, 123, 127

calcium channel-blockers, 171

California, 105, 131, 187

Canada, 22, 58, 174–75, 205n9

cancer: asymptomatic, 25, 26; as a chronic disease, 8; disparities in rates and kinds of, 63; drugs for, 11; screening for, 26; treatment centers for, 94. *See also* *specific kinds of cancer*

capitation, 38, 48, 75, 105, 136, 151

cardiovascular surgeons. *See* heart surgery

caregivers, 102, 104, 106

Care Management Performance Pilot Program, 123–24

care partnerships, 94, 95. *See also* teamwork

Caribbean immigrants, 61

"carve-outs," 75, 79

Casalino, Lawrence, 170

Casey, Robert, 137

Castro, Fidel, 61

cataracts, 116

CAT scans, 24, 26

CDHPs (consumer-driven health plans), 46–47

Celebrex (drug), 2, 3

Center for Patient Advocacy, 20

Centers for Medicare and Medicaid Services (CMS), 23, 105, 108, 122–24, 127, 131, 169

certification, 86–87, 153, 157–58

Chamber of Commerce, 15

Charter on Medical Professionalism, 157

Chassin, Mark, 21

chemical sensitivity disorders, 43

Chicago (Illinois), 51, 53

childbirth. *See* obstetrical care

children: insurance for, 37–38, 137, 161–64, 182, 185; medical care for, 88, 138–39; mental illness treatment for, 76, 78, 81, 133, 171, 198n26. *See also* infants

Children's Health Insurance Program, 37–38, 162, 163, 185

Chileans, 61

Chinese immigrants, 105

cholesterol (high), 41, 49, 52, 53, 118–19. *See also* statins

chronic disease (disabilities), 85, 186; challenges of, 8–10, 15, 100–101; comorbidity in, 9, 71, 78; consensus about, 161; costs associated with, 163; factors in, 64; and HSAs, 47; managing of, 156, 158, 169–70; and Medicaid, 182, 183, 185; studies of management of, 123–24. *See also* comorbidity; disease management programs; long-term care; *specific chronic diseases*

chronic fatigue syndrome, 41, 43

Cialis (drug), 131

cigarette smoking. *See* tobacco use

civic engagement. *See* social capital

civil servants, 57

class. *See* socioeconomic status

clinical pharmacists, 168

clinical trials. *See* randomized clinical trials

Clinton, Bill, 27, 106, 125–26, 159, 176, 179

CMS. *See* Centers for Medicare and Medicaid Services

Cochrane Collaboration, 97, 177

cognitive therapy, 74, 77

co-insurance, 46, 47. *See also* costs (of health care): sharing of

Columbia University Medical Center (New York City), 126

Commonwealth Fund, 23

communication, 70; as able to be taught, 151, 158; and gender, 186; among health agencies, 98, 127, 129, 157, 158; in hospitals, 10–11, 21, 27; between patients and physicians, 62, 78, 82, 84–85, 87, 92, 127, 128, 139, 143–44, 146, 150–51, 158. *See also* teamwork

community. *See* inequality; social capital (social fabric); trust

comorbidity, 9, 71, 78, 118, 199n32; among elderly, 101, 119–20

computerization: for chronic disease management, 169; to implement evidence-based medicine, 165; as increasing administrative costs, 175; of pharmaceutical information, 92; as quality-assurance tool, 10, 15, 18, 34, 98, 118, 127, 129, 158; as saving time, 49; in small practices, 96, 127, 168; in well-organized medical groups, 95. *See also* Internet; privacy

computerized axial tomography (CAT), 24

concierge medical practices, 93, 94

Congress (U.S.): on chronic disease management, 169–70; and Cox-2 inhibitors, 91; health groups' lobbying of, 20, 155; and Medicaid cutbacks, x; and Medicare, 33, 122, 131, 173; and nursing home quality, 107; on Patient's Bill of Rights, 153; trust in, 148. *See also* politics (of U.S. health care system); *specific legislation, committees, offices, and legislators*

Congressional Budget Office, 181

Congressional Office of Technology Assessment, 20

Connecticut, 103

Consumer Assessment of Health Plans Surveys (CAHPS), 123, 127

consumer-driven health plans (CDHPs), 46–47

"consumerism," 88–89. *See also* advertising; patient(s); profits

Consumers Union (CU), 91, 166

contraception, 63

contracts, 153–54

corporations: influence of, on U.S. health care system, ix, 1–3, 11–12, 14–15, 23, 25–26, 36, 97–99, 120; involvement of, in

definition of new diseases, 17, 25–26; political impact of, 3, 14, 81–82, 89–91, 172, 180. *See also* hospitals; insurance; medical devices: manufacturers of; pharmaceutical companies; profits

cosmetic surgery, 130, 135, 139

costs (of health care): administrative, 174–76; attempts to constrain, 1, 11–12, 15, 26, 27–28, 33, 45–48, 75–76, 94, 95, 104, 114–15, 127, 130–43, 162, 180–82; change often spurred by increased, 176; of comorbidity, 119; competition on basis of, 33, 89, 91, 92; and computerization, 96, 175; difficulties in constraining, 4–5, 25–26, 29, 37–38; insured patients as unaware of, 5, 22, 30–31, 85; for lifetime treatment of "new" diseases, 41; of long-term care, 101, 102, 106, 163; for Medicare and Medicaid, 12, 119, 163, 176, 180–85; of mental health treatment, 67, 81; new technology's contributions to, 23–26, 85, 87, 144; patients as unaware of, 5, 22, 30–31, 85; as percent of gross national product, 23, 29, 139; per person in the U.S., 20; physicians as unaware of, 91; of private Medicare Advantage Plans, 180; proportion of, paid by government, 23; rising, 23–24, 28, 29, 127, 163, 179; rising, drugs' role in, 11–12, 25–26, 41–42, 81–82, 90, 171, 172–73, 176; sharing of, 22, 23–24, 30, 45–46, 74–75, 174, 179, 181–84; for unnecessary and/or overused treatments, 5, 6, 11, 19–20, 24–25, 33, 34, 45, 48, 113, 165, 176–77. *See also* insurance (health); uninsured

coverage (insurance), 14, 160; and amount of medical use, 45, 117; gaps in continuity of, x, 6, 23, 133, 164; lack of long-term-care, in most insurance, 100, 102, 135; limits on, 6, 23, 28, 130–33, 141, 167; in Medicare D drug benefit, 11–12; parity, for mental health, 73; physicians as unaware of fine points of their patients,' 91; racial and ethnic disparities in, 60, 61; universal, ix, 6, 27, 48, 63. *See also* Children's Health Insurance Program; insurance; Medicaid; Medicare; uninsured persons

Cox-2 inhibitors, 1–3, 91, 153, 171–72
Cubans, 61

Daniels, Norman, 140
DARE (Drug Abuse Resistance Education), 81
Deal, Nathan, 131
death. *See* mortality
decision aids, 177–78
dementia, 100, 101–2, 104
Democratic Party, 22, 180
depression, 34, 40, 42, 48–50, 69, 72, 74;
    evidence-based treatments for, 76–78,
    198n29. *See also* antidepressants;
    Fluoxetine (drug); SSRIs
deprivation, 58, 59. *See also* inequality;
    poverty; social networks; socioeconomic
    status
"despairing optimists," 178
Deyo, Richard, 25
diabetes, 34, 48, 49, 123, 130
Diagnostic and Statistical Manual of the
    American Psychiatric Association (DSM-
    IV), 43, 67, 70–71, 80
dialysis, 134, 138
diet (nutrition): educating patients about,
    93; fortified food in, 63; as health risk, 7,
    36, 52, 56, 59, 63–65, 177; in long-term-
    care facilities, 101
disabilities. *See* chronic disease
disease advocacy groups, 15, 43, 50, 81–82,
    89, 139, 156. *See also* support groups;
    names of specific groups
disease management programs, 9, 34, 88,
    90, 95, 123, 165, 186; array of, 127; for
    chronic diseases, 49, 101, 123, 168–70;
    for depression, 78. *See also* teamwork
diseases, 39–50; Americans' lack of
    "fatalism" regarding, 22; asymptomatic,
    25, 26, 41–43, 49–50; controlling spread
    of, 21; cultural aspects of, 39–50;
    definitions of, 24, 39–50; environmental,
    social, and behavioral factors in, 7–8,
    36–37, 50, 52; global travel of, 12–13, 54;
    iatrogenic, 141; model for, 41; "new," 4,
    17, 24–25, 39–50, 67, 68, 93; number of
    people suffering from, 44; objective
    measures vs. subjective reports of, 43–45;
    patients with serious, 149–50, 152, 174;

prevention of, 1, 13, 17, 20, 21, 40, 53,
    56, 63, 88, 90, 93, 123, 188; race-linked,
    55; some, as self-limiting, 71, 72, 176.
    See also chronic disease; disease
    advocacy groups; disease management
    programs; health; medicalization;
    patient(s); physicians; *specific diseases*
"disrupted trust," 152–54
Doctor's Office Quality Project, 123
Dole, Bob, 130
"doughnut hole" (in Medicare Part D),
    11–12
Drug Abuse Resistance Education (DARE),
    81
drug detail representatives. *See* drugs:
    promotion of, to physicians
drugs (pharmaceutical): authority to
    prescribe, 76, 186; bargaining over price
    of, 12, 97, 173, 180; beneficial results
    from new, 52, 77; consumer information
    on, 91; errors in use of, 10, 170; as
    excluded from many insurance plans, 6,
    23, 82, 135, 183; formularies for, 48, 76,
    82, 90, 92, 133, 135, 171; generic, 90,
    172; increasing use of, 11, 68, 77;
    interactions of, 49, 92, 119, 170;
    "lifestyle," 131, 133; for mental illness,
    68, 75, 76–77, 80; "me-too," 91, 172, 173;
    new, as leading to new diseases, 4, 24,
    43, 93; new, as no more effective than
    old, 77, 84, 90, 91, 172, 173; in nursing
    homes, 107–8; patients' demand for
    certain, 2–3, 12, 18, 84, 92, 95, 131–32,
    172; promotion of, to physicians, 1, 2–3,
    77, 89–92, 97–98, 172, 173–74;
    regulation of, 90, 153, 160, 171; research
    needed on comparative effectiveness of,
    33, 91, 96–97, 165, 166, 172, 174;
    research on, as biased, 82, 84, 97–98,
    198n26; and rising health costs, 11–12,
    25–26, 81–82, 90, 171, 172–73, 176; role
    of, in rising health care costs, 11–12,
    25–26, 41–42, 81–82, 90, 171, 172–73,
    176; withdrawal of, from market, 1–3, 91,
    153, 171–72. *See also* advertising;
    pharmaceutical companies; profits;
    substance abuse; treatments; *specific*
    drugs and kinds of drugs
DSM-IV, 43, 67, 70–71, 80

DTC advertising. *See* advertising: direct-to-consumer drug
Dubos, René, 178
Dunedin (New Zealand), 40
dyspepsia, 116

ectopic pregnancies, 136
ED (erectile dysfunction) drugs, 82, 130–32, 139
Eden Alternative, 111
education, 66; continuing, for physicians, 89, 158, 172, 174; for evidence-based medicine, 167; of medical specialists, 86; and mental illness, 133; of patients, 33–34, 49, 92, 95, 124–26, 156, 168, 170, 177–78; of primary care physicians, 196n6; quality of U.S. medical, 20, 34; about sex, 63; and socioeconomic status, 55, 57–61; for women, 13, 65. *See also* certification; information; nursing schools; residents (medical)
elderly: abuse of, 107, 110, 112; comorbidity among, 101, 119–20; consensus on medical resources for, 161; costs associated with care for, 163, 185; not enough physicians to care for, 100; long-term care of, 9, 14, 15, 100–112, 135, 144; and private managed-care plans, 181; women as caregivers for, 102, 104, 106. *See also* Medicaid; Medicare; retirees
electronic medical records. *See* computerization
emergency rooms, 23, 162
employment status (of uninsured), 6, 163, 209n4
Endovascular Technologies, 3
England, 51, 53, 163. *See also* United Kingdom
enhancement drugs, 82, 93, 130–32, 139
entitlement programs. *See* Medicaid; Medicare; Social Security program
environment, 7, 13, 36, 40–50, 54–56, 59, 60, 64, 66
episiotomies, 25
erectile dysfunction drugs, 82, 130–32, 139
errors (medical): attempts to reduce, x, 15, 18, 94, 98, 156, 158, 160, 162; causes of, 115–16, 141, 170; in hospitals, 10–11, 21, 27, 34–35, 94, 100, 187; number of

annual, 116; number of drug, 170. *See also* litigation (over medical issues)
ethics (medical), 153, 157, 158; pharmaceutical companies' questionable, 3–4, 32, 81–82, 89, 90–91, 97–98, 155, 171–74, 198n26. *See also* accountability; professionalism (medical); research; trust
ethnicity, 55, 118; as factor in inequality of health care services, ix, 6–7, 60–63, 162. *See also specific ethnic groups*
Europe, 86, 90, 157; mortality and socioeconomic status in, 54–55, 63. *See also specific countries in*
European Federation of Internal Medicine, 157
evidence-based medicine, 11, 15, 18, 48, 49, 69, 95, 97, 113; as curtailing unnecessary and/or overused treatments, 5, 6, 11, 19–20, 24–25, 33, 34, 38, 45, 48, 113, 135–37, 141, 165, 176–77; defined, 115; medical care not usually based on, 5, 32, 76–77; in Medicare, 33; for mental illness treatment, 76–78; need for, 25, 164–67, 176–78; quality care enhanced by, 115, 118–20, 127; for rationing of health care, 140–41; studies of, 19–20, 32–34, 120, 123; in the UK, 32–33, 96–97, 165. *See also* randomized clinical trials
exercise, 7, 8, 52, 56, 93, 101, 177
exploitation (as a health issue), 13

Families USA, 15
FDA. *See* Food and Drug Administration
Federal Employees Health Benefits (FEHB) Program, 37, 73, 181
Federal Reserve, 165
fee-for-service medicine, 22, 25, 28, 35, 38, 44, 45, 48, 74–76, 85, 181
fetal-cell therapy, 25
Finland, 53
Fisher, Elliott, 25
flexible spending plans, 29
fluoridation (of water), 63
Fluoxetine (drug), 140–41, 198nn29, 31
folic acid, 42
Food and Drug Administration (FDA), 82; change in research approach needed by, 97, 172; drug industry as helping to fund, 3, 90–91, 171; as drug regulator, 90,

Food and Drug Administration (FDA)
  (continued)
  153, 171; lack of post-marketing drug
  studies by, 3, 91, 171
foster care facilities, 101, 103, 106, 110,
  112. *See also* long-term care
France, 205n11
full-body screening, 24, 26

gastrointestinal problems, 1–2, 45
gender: and communication, 186; as factor
  in inequality of health care services, 17;
  as factor in treatment plans, 118–19. *See
  also* men; women
General Electric, 129
General Motors Corporation, 129
general practice physicians (GPs). *See*
  primary care physicians
geographical region: as factor in inequality
  of health care services, ix, 6–7, 11, 17,
  134, 142; medical service availability in,
  62, 63, 132, 181, 186; psychiatric service
  availability in, 76, 132–33
Germany, 205n11
gerontologists, 100
Gittelsohn, Alan, 117
government (U.S.), 26; American distrust of
  big, 162; and decision aids, 178; and
  drug-price bargaining, 12, 97, 173, 180;
  erosion of trust in, 3–4, 22, 35, 147–48,
  155; as guaranteeing savings accounts,
  153; need for standards by, to protect
  patients, 4, 32–34; policy of, on health
  disparities, 60, 113; rationing of ED
  drugs by, 130–32; responsibility of, for
  mentally ill, 80–81, 83; subsidies by, for
  employer-sponsored insurance, 23, 29;
  subsidies for national health information
  network needed from, 165; subsidies to
  hospitals from, 162. *See also* Congress;
  taxes; United States; *specific agencies,
  programs, and presidents of*
Grassley, Charles, 131
Great Britain. *See* United Kingdom
Green, Larry, 44
Greenberg, Bernard, 44
Green House Project, 111–12
Group Health Cooperative of Puget Sound
  (Washington), 156, 169

group homes (for the elderly), 103, 106
Guidant (company), 3
guns, 36, 63, 65

"Harry and Louise" (television ads), 159
Harvard Medical School, 84, 119
Haught, Randall, 29–30
headaches, 45, 143
health: care for, as a "right," 22; consensus
  on good, 161; as a continuum, 41;
  definitions of, 24, 69; environmental,
  social, and behavioral factors affecting,
  7–8, 13, 36–37, 50, 52; medical care only
  a small part of forces that shape, 36,
  51–52; as part of larger culture, 1, 51–66;
  promotion of, 1, 13, 17, 20, 21, 40, 53,
  56, 63, 88, 90, 93, 123, 188; promotion
  of, in long-term care system, 9, 101; self-
  assessment of, 69–70; U.S.'s scores on
  indicators of, ix–x, 6, 20, 115, 141, 188.
  See also diet; diseases; exercise;
  population health; public health; risks
Health and Human Services Department, 33
Health Canada, 22
health care proxies, 10
health care system (U.S.): attempts to fix, as
  creating new problems, x, 120, 125, 126,
  154; consensus on issues regarding,
  161–62; corporate influence as skewing
  patient service in, ix, 1–3, 11–12, 14–15,
  23, 25–26, 36, 97–99, 120; "dynamics
  without change" characterization of, 37;
  financing of, 14, 17, 25–26, 37, 38, 74,
  117, 162; fragmented nature of, 8–9, 20,
  27, 87, 147, 162, 170; goals of ideal, 48;
  how to reshape, to function better for
  patients, x; impact of American values
  on, 1, 5, 15, 17, 22, 23, 30, 60, 159, 162,
  164, 180; inequality in, ix, 6–7, 17, 20,
  46–48, 56–57, 60, 93, 94, 135, 141, 142,
  157, 160–62, 182, 188; as a non-system,
  20, 38, 39–40; polarization of views of,
  13–14, 22–23, 37, 182; politics of, 14–15,
  19–20, 32–33, 37–38, 96, 123, 124,
  130–32, 135–37, 155, 159–60, 164, 172,
  181; public views of, 159; range of
  choices in, for insured, 20, 22; reform
  possibilities for, 19–38, 159–82. *See also*
  chronic disease; costs; coverage;

diseases; errors (medical); hospitals;
inequality; insurance; long-term care;
medicine; nurses; patient(s); physicians;
quality; rationing; trust
health maintenance organizations (HMOs),
27, 28, 33, 105, 136, 140, 147, 155, 168,
186; administrative costs of large, 175;
drug purchasing by, 173; mental illness
treatment by, 75; surveys of, 156–57. *See
also* managed care
Health Partners (Minnesota), 156
Health Plan Data and Information Set
(HEDIS), 124–25, 127
Health Savings Account (HSA), 46–47, 144
heart attacks (myocardial infarction):
attempts to prevent, 41, 42; contributions
to, 2, 58; incidence of, 53; quality of care
for, 31, 122
heart disease (cardiovascular disease), 81,
130; as a chronic disease, 8; decline in
mortality from, 52; drugs for, 11; gender
factors in, 118–19; national differences in
levels of, 53; quality of treatment of, 122,
123
heart failure, 31, 34, 49, 119, 122, 123
heart surgery (cardiovascular surgery), 33,
52, 87, 125–26, 155
HEDIS (Health Plan Data and Information
Set), 124–25, 127
Hevesi, Alan, 131
hierarchy (and health). *See* autonomy
hip surgery, 31, 116, 122
"Hispanic paradox," 195n25
Hispanics, 55, 60, 61, 195n25
HIV. *See* AIDS
HMOs. *See* health maintenance organizations
H5N1 virus (avian flu virus), 13, 54
home care (for the elderly), 102–6, 110, 112
homicide, 51, 53, 58
homosexuality, 39, 67
hormone replacement therapy, 26
hospice, 9–10
hospitalists, x
Hospital Quality Incentive Demonstration
Project, 122–24
hospitals: advertising of, 152; antibiotic-
resistant infections in, 13; attempts to
improve quality of treatments in,

122–24; as developing around new
techniques and medical approaches, 25;
economic rather than medical reasons
for stays in, 75, 117; emergency rooms
of, 23, 162; errors in, 10–11, 21, 27,
34–35, 94, 100, 187; government
subsidies to, 162; impact of Medicare's
PPS on, 120, 173; infrastructures of U.S.,
20; and managed care, 27; nurses in,
186–87; psychiatric, 68, 75, 76, 79, 80,
109, 154; quality-of-care data on, 31, 33,
125–27, 141, 145; quality of death in, 10;
specialized, 155. *See also* nurses;
physicians; teamwork
House Ways and Means Committee, 106
housing, 55, 59
HRT (hormone replacement therapy), 26
HSAs (Health Savings Account), 46–47, 144
human capital, 65
hypertension (high blood pressure), 41–42,
48–49, 52–53, 56, 123, 199n32; drugs for,
41, 48, 52, 91
hypochondriacs, 44, 68–69
hyzdralazine (BiDil), 119

ICDs (implantable cardioverter-defibrillators), 3
ideology. *See* United States: impact of
values of, on health care system
"illness behavior," 43, 61–62
immigrants, 6–8, 61, 105. *See also specific
racial, ethnic, and national groups*
immunizations, 48, 88, 93
implantable cardioverter-defibrillators
(ICDs), 3
inactivity. *See* exercise
income: consensus about medical care and,
161; and government insurance
eligibility, 163; of medical specialists, 87,
88; and mental illness, 133; of nursing
home staff, 109–10; of physicians, 24, 27,
50, 87, 88, 93, 95, 127, 167–68, 181, 185,
186, 188; of primary care physicians, 87,
167, 168; redistributing, 57, 60, 124; and
socioeconomic status, 55, 57–60. *See
also* employment status; occupations;
poverty; wages vs. benefits
India, 61
Industry Profile, 89–90

inequality (in U.S. health care system), ix, 6–7, 17, 20, 46–48, 56–57; American tolerance of, 141, 142; concierge care as contributing to, 93, 94; future, in Medicare, 182; implicit rationing and, 135; opposition to, 157, 161–62, 188; reduction of, 160; not solely a cause of poor health, 60

infants, 51–52, 55, 56, 61, 62

influenza pandemics, 13, 54

information: conflicting, on health, 14, 24, 35, 115, 145; about health plans, 88–89, 125–27; on hospital quality, 31–32, 47; on Internet, 89, 93, 125–27, 145, 150, 156, 177; on medical costs, 47; need for unbiased, 97, 165, 172, 174, 177; on nursing home quality, 33, 108; overwhelming amount of, 93, 97, 107, 120, 127–28; patients' gathering of, 85, 107, 134, 150, 155–56, 177; pharmaceutical, from physicians, 91, 172; and socioeconomic status, 56–57. See also advertising; disease advocacy groups; education; evidence-based medicine; media; patient support groups; research

information technologies. See computerization

informed consent, 153, 154

Institute for Geriatric Nursing (New York University), 110

Institute of Medicine (IOM), 19, 107, 116, 165–66, 204n27

institutional review boards, 153

insurance (health): cost constraint pressures vs. patients' demands on, 4–6, 45–46, 73–76, 85, 167; excluded treatments in most, 6, 23, 73, 74–77, 82, 100, 102, 133, 135, 183; lack of universal, in U.S., 6, 15, 22, 27–28, 38, 161, 174–76; for long-term care, 100, 102–3, 135, 144; orientation of, to episodic acute situations rather than chronic disease, 8, 102, 169; parity for mental health coverage in, 73; and pay-for-performance programs, 9, 129; payment of, in U.S., 5, 23, 29–30; persons with, loath to accept changes in, 159; physicians' dealings with, 91, 93–94; plans for, 14, 31, 33–34, 38, 46, 75, 82, 88–89, 93, 96, 97, 120–21, 125,

133, 140, 168, 178, 180–81; proposals for universal, 27–28, 161–63, 188; quality of care variations with, 76; rating of various plans for, 125, 126; requiring individuals to purchase private, 162; some elements of universal, available in U.S., x, 37; universal coverage by, in most developed countries, ix, 6, 27, 48. See also Children's Health Insurance Program; co-insurance; costs; coverage (insurance); managed care; Medicaid; Medicare; pay-for-performance programs; reimbursement; underinsured persons; uninsured persons; wages vs. benefits

internal mammary artery ligation, 25

International Classification of Disease, 71

Internet, 25; health information on, 89, 93, 125–27, 145, 150, 156, 177

interpersonal skills. See communication

interpersonal therapy, 74, 77

"interpersonal trust," 149–51

in vitro fertilization, 139

IOM. See Institute of Medicine

Iraq War, 159

isosorbide dinitrate, 119

Jacobs, Lawrence, 136

jails. See prison system (U.S.)

JAMA. See Journal of the American Medical Association

Japan, 53

John A. Hartford Foundation, 110

Johns Hopkins Medical School, 152

Joint Commission on Accreditation of Healthcare Organizations (JCAHO), 31

Journal of the American Medical Association (JAMA), 82, 90, 91, 98, 171

Kaiser Foundation Health Plan, 15

Kaiser Permanente Medical Groups, 95, 118, 120, 141, 156, 175, 181

Kane, Rosalie, 111–12

King, Steven, 131

Klein, Rudolf, 131, 132

knee surgery, 25, 31, 122

laminectomies, 19

The Lancet, 26, 82, 90, 98

language difficulties, 60, 61

lead exposure, 56, 65
LeapFrog Group, 129
leukemia, 137, 138–39
Levitra (drug), 131
life-care communities, 104
"lifestyle drugs," 131, 133
Link, Bruce, 56–57, 63
litigation (over medical issues), 1–3, 64, 135, 138–40, 147, 149, 153–54, 167, 188, 206n28
living wills, 10
long-term care, 9, 14, 15, 100–112, 135, 144, 182, 184, 185. *See also* nursing homes
low density lipoproteins, 42
lung cancer, 26, 63
Lyme disease, 43

magnetic resonance imaging (MRIs), 24, 143
Magnuson, Warren, 138
malpractice. *See* errors (medical); litigation
mammography, 26
managed care: as attempt to control health costs, 27–28, 48, 136, 143, 181; backlash against, 5, 27–28, 86, 132, 135, 151, 153; as demand on physicians' time, 94; for mental illness, 74, 75–77, 79; rationing by, 5. *See also* health maintenance organizations
Mantle, Mickey, 137
Mariel (Cuba), 61
marketing. *See* advertising
markets. *See* profits
Marmot, Michael, 57
mastectomies, 25, 153
masturbation, 39
Mayo Clinic, 151, 152
McClellan, Mark, 131
Mechanic, David: IOM pain committee chaired by, 19; and Institute for Geriatric Nursing, 110; HMO study by, 156–57; research on mental illness by, 106, 109; and Ticket to Work program, 106; at University of Washington Medical School, 137–38; and U.S. Advisory Committee on Vital and Health Statistics, 108
media: direct-to-consumer drug advertising in, 1–3, 12, 14, 25, 35, 77, 81, 84, 89–91, 93, 118, 130–31, 145, 150, 171, 173, 174; feelings of deprivation elicited by, 59; on

HMOs, 28; information supplied by, 34, 145, 156, 166, 177, 188; mental illness depicted in, 71; trust and social fabric undermined by, 35–36, 114, 147, 154, 156, 159, 166. *See also* advertising; Internet
Medicaid, 14; children's coverage by, 163; costs of, 12, 119, 163, 176, 180–85; drug purchasing by, 173; dual enrollees of, with Medicare, 12, 105, 183–85; federal role in, 23, 30, 37, 103, 180, 182–84; growth in, 30, 180; impending financial crisis in, 12, 144, 180–85; limitations on coverage by, 1, 131, 133, 135–37; for long-term care of the destitute, 102, 103–4, 108–9, 182, 184, 185; for mental illness treatment, 68, 75, 79, 81, 184; number of people covered by, 182; pharmaceutical companies' lobbying of, 90; proposals for changes in, x, 162, 180, 184–85; state role in, 12, 30, 68, 79, 108, 131, 135–37, 182; variation in, from state to state, 79, 103–4, 108, 163, 182–84. *See also* taxes
medical devices: insurance as excluding, 23; manufacturers of, 3, 19, 25, 32; testing of, 90, 166. *See also* technology (new)
medical education. *See* education
Medical Expenditure Panel Survey, 44
medicalization (of normal problems of living), 4, 24, 39–50, 70, 82. *See also* diseases: "new"
medical records (computerized). *See* computerization
medical savings accounts. *See* Health Savings Account
Medicare, 14; and computerization, 98; costs of, 12, 119, 163, 175, 176, 180–85; 2006 drug benefit in, 11–12, 23, 107, 131, 170, 173, 176, 180, 184; drug-price bargaining not permitted by, 12, 97, 173, 180; dual enrollees of, with Medicaid, 12, 105, 183–85; evidence-based medicine in, 33; federal role in, 22, 23, 33, 37, 68, 180–84; impending financial crisis in, 29, 180–82; limitations on coverage by, 1, 131, 133; mental illness treatment through, 68; pay-for-performance initiatives in, 11,

Medicare (continued)
122–24; PPS plan in, 48, 120; proposals
for changes in, x, 162, 164, 180; racial
disparities in, 61–62; as single-payer
health insurance, 22; taxes for, 29, 30
Medicare Advantage Plans, 180
Medicare Modernization Act (MMA). See
Medicare Prescription Drug, Improvement and Modernization Act (2003)
Medicare Part D (2006), 11–12, 23, 107,
131, 170, 176, 184
Medicare Prescription Drug, Improvement,
and Modernization Act (2003), 33, 34,
123–24, 169, 180
medicine: alternative and complementary,
17, 68, 83, 177; care in, not generally
evidence-based, 5, 32, 76–77;
decentralized nature of, in U.S., 12, 32,
112, 152, 168, 174–75; defensive, 154,
206n28; erosion of trust in, 3–4, 143–58;
fee-for-service, 22, 25, 28, 35, 38, 44, 45,
48, 74–76, 85, 181; as fragmented and
specialized, 8–9, 27, 32, 86–88, 147, 162,
170; as marketable product, 22, 88–89;
need for evidence-based, 25; as part of
larger culture, 1, 22–23, 39–66;
preventive, 1, 13, 17, 20, 21, 40, 53, 56,
63, 88, 90, 93, 123, 188; specialties and
subspecialties in, 4, 9; standards for
evidence-based, 19–20, 32–34, 120, 123;
traditional practice of, 84–85, 128;
uncertainty in, 2, 5, 19, 25, 26, 34, 35,
90, 115, 118, 150. See also costs;
diseases; drugs; evidence-based
medicine; health; hospitals; inequality;
insurance; litigation; nurses; patient(s);
pharmaceutical companies; physicians;
population health; public health; science;
specialists; technology; treatments
men, 52, 118–19
mental illness, 14, 67–83, 126; in children,
76, 78, 81, 133, 171, 198n26; and
comorbidity, 199n32; costs of treating,
67, 81; deinsitutionalization of those
with serious, 79–81; drugs for, 11, 76–78;
exclusion of care for, in many insurance
plans, 6, 23, 73, 74–77, 133, 135, 183;
fragmentation of services for those
suffering from, 79; imprisoning of

persons suffering from, 68, 80, 81;
meanings of, 67; medically relevant, vs.
adjustment issues, 73–74; numbers of
people suffering, 70–72, 197n16; serious
and persistent, 71–72, 74, 76–77, 79–81,
83, 133, 184; and socioeconomic status,
133; stigmatization of persons with, 50;
treatment of, as government responsibility, 80–81, 83; types of need and care
for, 77, 198n26; variety of practitioners
in field of, 68, 74, 76. See also specific
mental illnesses
mental institutions. See hospitals:
psychiatric
Merck & Co., 2
Mexican Americans, 55, 60, 61, 195n25
Minnesota, 111, 156, 170
Mississippi, 103, 111–12
Mor, Vincent, 109
morality, 130, 131. See also ethics; religion
Mormons, 65–66
Morone, James A., 66
mortality (death): corporate responsibility
for some, 2, 3; declines in, from heart
disease, 52, 119; due to medical error, 10,
27, 34, 116; environmental, social, and
behavioral factors in, 7–8, 52; hospital
data regarding, 126; of infants, 51–52, 55,
56, 61, 62; medical care as having
limited influence on, 51–52; need to
reduce U.S., 20; nurse-patient ratios in
hospitals related to, 186–87; in nursing
homes, 9–10, 100; racial and ethnic
factors in, 60–62, 195n25; reduction in,
associated with strong primary care, 88;
and socioeconomic status, 23, 54–60;
among uninsured, 23, 162, 190n8; U.S.'s
scores on indicators of, ix–x, 6, 20, 115,
141, 188. See also diseases; suicide
MRIs, 24, 143
murder. See homicide
Muslims, 65
myocardial infarction. See heart attacks

naproxen (drug), 1, 2
National Academy of Sciences, 165–66,
204n27
National Alliance for the Mentally Ill, 15,
43, 74

National Committee for Quality Assurance (NCQA), 124–25, 204n27

National Comorbidity Study, 71, 72

National Governors Association, 184, 185

National Health Service (NHS—UK), 33, 86, 96–97, 120–22, 124, 126, 134–35, 168, 176

National Institute for Health and Clinical Excellence (NICE–UK), 32–33, 96–97, 165

National Institutes of Health, 97, 173

National Opinion Research Corporation, 143–44

National Quality Forum (2003), 11

Native Americans, 60

neurasthenia, 69

neurologists, 87

New England Journal of Medicine, 2, 82, 89, 90, 98, 116–17, 179

New Freedom Initiative, 106, 107

New York, 103, 110, 126, 131

New York University, 110

NHS. *See* National Health Service (UK)

NICE. *See* National Institute for Health and Clinical Excellence

No Free Lunch (professional health group), 174

North American Spine Society, 20

nurse practitioners, 34, 76, 85, 112, 129, 168, 186

nurses: and chronic care patients, 9, 168; for nursing homes, 110, 132; psychiatric, 76; as relieving physicians' workload, 49, 85; shortage of, x, 132, 186–87. *See also* nurse practitioners; teamwork

nurses' aides, 109–10

nursing homes: amount of care in, paid by Medicaid, 103; benefits of, 104, 107, 110; elderly people's fear of, 103, 110; end-of-life issues in, 9–10, 100; number of people in, 107; problems with community alternatives to, 107, 110, 112; quality of care in, 101, 107–8; quality-of-care information on, 33, 108; staff at, 108–10, 112, 132, 186; standards for, 108, 110; use of, to reduce hospital costs, 120. *See also* long-term care

nursing schools, 110

nutrition. *See* diet

obesity, 7, 49, 64

obsessive-compulsive disorders, 72

obstetrical care, 25, 31, 48, 88, 89, 153. *See also* ectopic pregnancies

obstructive pulmonary disease, 123

occupations, 55, 57, 59, 61. *See also* employment status; income; wages vs. benefits

office staff (in physicians' offices), 94, 123

OHP (Oregon Health Plan), 135–37, 139

Oklahoma, 103

Olmstead v. L.C., 103–4

Omnibus Budget Reconciliation Act (1986), 105

Omnibus Budget Reconciliation Act (1987), 108

On-Lok, 104

Oregon, 103, 135–37, 139

Oregon Health Plan (OHP), 135–37, 139

Organization for Economic Co-operation and Development (OECD), 6

orthopedic surgeons, 19–20, 155

osteoarthritis, 123

Overdosed America (Abramson), 84

PACE (Program of All Inclusive Care for the Elderly), 105

Pacific Business Group on Health, 129

PACT (Program for Assertive Community Treatment), 79

pain, 10, 19–20, 43–44, 49

pancreatic cancer, 63

panic disorder, 72. *See also* anxiety

paperwork costs, 174–76

paranoia, 149

Parkinson's disease, 25

Parsons, Talcott, 84

partnerships (for care), 94, 95. *See also* teamwork

patient(s): changing role of, 14, 84–99; corporate influence as skewing service to, ix, 1–3, 11–12, 14–15, 23, 25–26, 36, 97–99, 120; cost constraint pressures on insurance vs. demands of, 4–6, 45–46, 73–76, 85, 167; decreased attention to whole, x, 8–10, 21, 88, 167; demands of, for new drugs and treatments, 2–3, 12, 18, 26, 35–36, 84–99, 123–24, 134, 135, 140, 141, 156, 167, 169, 176–78; educating,

Patient(s) *(continued)*
  33–34, 49, 92, 95, 124–26, 156, 168, 170,
  177–78; friends and relatives as
  influences on, 34, 125, 146, 149, 150,
  177; how to reshape health care system
  so that it functions better for, x;
  information-gathering by, 85, 107, 134,
  150, 155–56, 177; perceptions of disease
  by, 43–44; physician characteristics
  valued by, 127, 150–51; physicians as
  making choices for, 34, 46, 47, 90;
  privacy of, 98, 153; as receiving less or
  more than recommended amount of care,
  116–17; as seeking a medical fix rather
  than a healthy lifestyle, 176–77; surveys
  of medical experiences of, 123, 127; tools
  to heighten trust among, 157; trust of, in
  their personal physicians, 34, 35, 91,
  114, 125, 143–46, 148–50, 156, 177, 178;
  as unable to navigate health care system,
  27; as unaware of medical costs, 5, 22,
  30–31, 85; as unwilling to accept
  limitations on care, 5, 17, 30–31, 35–36,
  84, 132, 138–40, 164–65, 177. *See also*
  communication; quality (of care);
  rationing; support groups; *specific
  diseases*
Patient's Bill of Rights, 153
patient support groups, 43, 82, 89, 169. *See
  also* disease advocacy groups
Patrick, Donald, 25
Payer, Lynn, 205n11
pay-for-performance programs, 9, 119–21,
  123–26, 128–29, 141, 165, 176; in
  Medicare, 11, 122–24
"pay or play," 162
PCPs. *See* primary care physicians
peer pressure, 7, 8
performance. *See* pay-for-performance
  programs; quality (of care)
pernicious anemia, 41
Peru, 41
PET scans, 24
pharmaceutical companies, 4; amount of
  money spent on advertising by, 89–91,
  96, 173; as defining new diseases for
  their drugs, 4, 43; direct-to-consumer
  drug advertising by, 1–3, 12, 14, 25, 35,
  77, 81, 84, 89–91, 93, 118, 130–31, 145,
  171, 173, 174; and drug formularies, 82,
  92, 104; drug research by, 97–98; ethical
  issues involving, 1–4, 32, 81–82, 89–91,
  97–98, 155, 171–74, 198n26; and 2006
  Medicare drug benefit, 11–12, 173, 176,
  180; and mental illness, 81–82; promotion of drugs to physicians by, 1, 2–3,
  77, 89–92, 97–98, 172, 173–74; stakes of,
  in marketing new drugs, 25, 32, 81–82;
  subsidies to, 173, 176, 180. *See also*
  drugs; profits
Pharmaceutical Research and Manufacturers of America, 89
pharmacists (clinical), 168
Phelan, Jo, 56–57, 63
phen-fen (drug), 171
PhRMA, 89
physician assistants, 76, 85, 129, 168, 186
physicians: accountability of, 21, 108, 118,
  129, 158; autonomy of, 27–28, 127, 135,
  140, 156, 164–65; as center of patient
  care, 21, 36; certification of, 86–87, 153,
  157–58; changing role of, 14, 49, 84–99,
  128–29; characteristics of, valued by
  patients, 127, 150–51; concierge
  practices of some, 93, 94; conflicts of
  interest of, 90, 153, 155, 158, 172,
  173–74; drugs promoted to, 1, 2–3, 77,
  89–92, 97–98, 172, 173–74; implicit
  rationing as permitting bias in service by,
  135; incomes of, 24, 27, 50, 87, 88, 93,
  95, 127, 167–68, 181, 185, 186, 188;
  individuals' right to choose their own,
  22, 27, 105, 149, 156, 157; as making
  choices for their patients, 34, 46, 47, 90;
  and managed care, 27–28; medical
  devices marketed to, 3; need for more, in
  long-term care, 100, 110; and nurses,
  187; office staff of, 94, 123; patients
  demanding new drugs and treatments
  from, 2–3, 12, 18, 26, 35–36, 84–99,
  123–24, 134, 135, 140, 141, 156, 167,
  169, 176–78; patients' trust in their
  personal, 34, 35, 91, 114, 125, 143–46,
  148–50, 156, 177, 178; and pay-for-
  performance schemes, 121; in small
  practices, 95–96, 120, 123, 127, 129, 156,
  168; supply and financing of, as affecting
  quality of service by, 117; time

constraints on, 35, 49, 77, 78, 87, 91, 92–95, 127, 165, 172; treatment of dying patients by, 9–10; women as, 168, 186. *See also* communication; medicine; primary care physicians; professionalism (medical); professional medical groups; quality (of care); reimbursement; specialists; teamwork

Picker Institute, 127

placebo effect, 70, 77, 97, 172, 176

pneumonia, 31, 122

politics (of U.S. health care system), 14–15, 19–20, 32–33, 37–38, 96, 123, 124, 130–32, 135–37, 155, 159–60, 164, 172, 181

polypills, 42, 53

Poor Laws (England), 163

population health, 7–8, 14–15, 17, 21, 36–37, 44–45, 51–66, 88, 118, 160, 170. *See also* public health

positron emission tomography (PET), 24

poverty: consensus on, 162; as health issue, 13, 57; increase in, in U.S., 185; long-term-care coverage for those in, 100; of nursing home staff, 109–10; programs targeted toward those in, 60. *See also* income; socioeconomic status; underinsured persons; uninsured persons

PPS. *See* prospective payment systems

practice guidelines. *See* evidence-based medicine: studies of

prenatal care, 116. *See also* obstetrical care

prepaid organized health practices, 95, 156, 168, 169, 175, 181. *See also* health maintenance organizations; Kaiser Permanente Medical Groups

President's New Freedom Commission on Mental Health, 80

"Prevention Paradox," 54

primary care physicians (PCPs), 94, 196n6; of African American patients, 62; in England, 121–22, 135; as guides through treatment and rehabilitation, 8–9, 85, 88, 152; and hospitalists, x; incomes of, 87, 167, 168; mental illness treatment by, 72, 73, 76–79, 82; need for more, 86–88, 167–68, 186; as referring patients to specialists, 27, 45, 48, 73, 78, 85, 86, 94, 133, 134, 152; role of, 85–86

"primary relationships," 146, 149

prison system (U.S.), 28, 131, 139; mentally ill incarcerated in, 68, 80, 81

privacy, 98, 153

privatization, 12, 47–48, 107, 180–81

Prizm 2 DR (ICD), 3

professionalism (medical), 95, 97, 99, 128–29, 151, 157–58, 173–74

professional medical groups: attempts to win public's trust by, 157–58, 173–74; conflicts of interest of, with drug and device manufacturers, 32, 89–90, 98–99; decentralization of, in U.S., 1, 14, 35, 96, 147, 155; of medical subspecialties as private organizations, 86; need to change, 14; political lobbying by, 20, 23–24, 124, 139, 181; public's distrust of, 35, 114. *See also* medicine; physicians; professionalism; *specific medical groups*

profits: emphasis on, as American value, 1; emphasis on, in medicine, 22; influence of corporate, on U.S. health care system, ix, 2–3, 12, 14–15, 17, 50, 97–99, 155, 172, 188; of pharmaceutical industry, 172–73; Ticket to Work program motivated by, 106–7. *See also* advertising (marketing)

Program for Assertive Community Treatment (PACT), 79

Program of All Inclusive Care for the Elderly (PACE), 105

prospective payment systems (PPS), 38, 48, 120, 181. *See also* Medicare

prostate cancer, 25, 26, 130

prostate-specific antigen (PSA) testing, 26, 177

Prozac (drug). *See* Fluoxetine (drug)

PSA testing, 26, 177

pseudodiseases, 25. *See also* diseases: asymptomatic

psychiatrists, 72–79, 132–33

psychoanalysis, 74

psychologists, 76–77

psychotherapy, 74–77

public "detailing," 96–97, 172

public health, 54, 56, 63–66, 136, 164. *See also* population health

Puerto Ricans, 61

Putnam, Robert D., 65

quality (of care), 115–29; for chronic diseases, 9–10, 170; communication as essential to, 70; competition on basis of, 33, 124–26; in emergency rooms, 23; enhancement of, by doing less, 113, 188; factors in, 117, 186–87; hospitalists vs. primary care physicians and, x; in long-term-care facilities, 101–2, 105, 108–10, 112; for mental illness, 76; need to raise, 11, 20, 34, 115–29, 162, 177; patient assessment of, 150; racial disparities in, 61–62; systems for implementing, 113–29, 141, 151–52, 160; transparency linked to, 31–32, 108. *See also* errors (medical); evidence-based medicine; mortality; patient(s); quality assurance programs
quality assurance programs, 10–11, 48, 93–95, 152, 158

race: as factor in inequality of health care services, ix, 6–7, 17, 20, 60–63, 109, 142, 161; as factor in treatment plans, 118, 119; and mortality, 60–63; and socioeconomic status, 55, 58
radical mastectomies, 25, 153
RAND Corporation, 116–17
randomized clinical trials (RCTs), 70, 177; for drugs, 26, 119; in evidence-based medicine, 115, 118, 119, 165, 176; limitations of, 166, 167
rationing (of health care), 14, 130–42; attempts at equitable, 15, 45–46; current, 132–33; for the elderly, 104; explicit vs. implicit, 5, 28, 134–37; lack of consensus about, 180; need for equitable, 34, 139–42; "tragic choices" in, 137–39; transparency needed in, 135, 139, 140; types of, 132
RCTs. *See* randomized clinical trials
reform possibilities (for health care system), 19–38, 159–82
regulation: difficulties with, 154, 175; of drugs, 90, 153, 171; by government, 97, 108, 112, 140; of health care rationing process, 140; as increasing trust, 152–54; of medical specialists, 86; of nursing homes, 108, 112; physicians' views of, 27; Republican views of, 22. *See also* quality (of care)

rehabilitation, 23, 101, 106
reimbursement: for elder care, 108–9, 112, 181; eligibility for, 74; to hospitals, 27, 120; influence of, on medical practice, 85, 155; linked to disease identification, 43; reduced, to physicians, 24, 27, 167, 181, 185, 188
religion, 10, 65–66. *See also* ethics; morality
Relman, Arnold, 179
Republican Party, 22, 46, 179–80
reputation (of physicians), 152
research (medical): on disease management, 169; ethical issues regarding, 1–4, 32, 81–82, 84, 90, 97–98, 124–25, 155, 166, 171–73, 198n26; evaluating quality of, 165, 166, 176; need for, on comparative effectiveness of drugs, 33, 91, 96–97, 165, 166, 172, 174; physicians' reputations often based on, 152; quality of U.S., 20, 34; on role of economics in provision of services, 117; volunteers for, 124, 153, 154. *See also* evidence-based medicine; pharmaceutical companies; randomized clinical trials; science
residence (and socioeconomic status), 55, 59
residents (medical), x, 158, 174
retirees, 164, 182
retirement communities (life-care communities), 104
risks: cultural aspects of, 42, 51–66; environmental, social, and behavioral, 7–8, 36–37, 55–56; of high blood pressure, 41; of homicide, 51, 53; individual vs. population, 2, 7–8, 36–37, 52–54; involved in trust, 145, 153; of new drugs, 91; of new technology, 45; of privatization of elder care, 107; undermining of concept of shared, 47–48
Robert Wood Johnson Foundation (RWJF), 102–3, 169
Roemer, Milton, 117
Roemer's Law, 117
Rose, Geoffrey, 52–54
Rosenthal, Marsha, 156–57
"rule of rescue," 136
RWJF (Robert Wood Johnson Foundation), 102–3, 169

Sabin, James, 140

Sackett, David, 115

safety net (U.S.), x, 79, 103. *See also* Medicaid; Medicare; State Children's Health Insurance Program

San Francisco (California), 105

SARS (Severe Acute Respiratory Syndrome), 13

savings accounts: financial, 152–53; for health care, 46–47, 144

SCHIP. *See* State Children's Health Insurance Program

schizophrenia, 71, 72, 74, 76, 137

Schwarzenegger, Arnold, 187

sciatica, 19

science: lack of, in DSM-IV, 43; lack of unbiased, regarding what is useful and what is wasteful, 19–20, 24, 34–35, 124–25; skepticism about, 166. *See also* evidence-based medicine; research

Science, 117

screening technologies, 24, 26

Scribner, Belding, 138

Scribner shunt, 138

seat belts (in automobiles), 63

"secondary relationships," 146, 151

secondhand smoke, 64. *See also* tobacco use

self-employment, 29

September 11, 2001 terrorist attack, 54

serotonin transporter (5-HT T) gene, 40

serotonin uptake inhibitors. *See* SSRIs

SES. *See* socioeconomic status

Severe Acute Respiratory Syndrome (SARS), 13

sexual behavior, 39, 93; drugs to enhance, 82, 130–32, 139; education about, 63; as a health risk, 13, 65

Sheils, John, 29–30

SHMO (Social Health Maintenance Organization), 105–6

slavery, 7

smoking. *See* tobacco use

social capital (social fabric), 35–36, 54, 57, 65, 89, 142, 149–51. *See also* inequality; trust

social class (defined), 55. *See also* socioeconomic status

social health, 69, 166

Social Health Maintenance Organization (SHMO), 105–6

social networks, 7, 65–66, 101

Social Security program, 12, 29, 180, 185

The Social Transformation of American Medicine (Starr), 147

"social trust," 151–52, 156

social workers, 9, 75–77

socioeconomic status (SES), ix, 6–7, 17, 54–60, 63, 142, 161. *See also* income; poverty

soldiers, 44

South Carolina, 103

spas, 133, 135, 205n11

special interests. *See* corporations; disease advocacy groups; hospitals; pharmaceutical companies; physicians; professional medical groups; specialists

specialists (physicians): chronic care management by, 9; competition among, 147, 155; as developing around new techniques and medical approaches, 4, 25, 32, 43, 87; in England, 168; in Europe, 86; incomes of, 24, 27, 50, 87, 88, 93, 95, 127, 167–68, 181, 185, 186, 188; patient demand for, 134; primary care offered by, 85, 86, 88; quality-of-care information about, 33; referrals to, 27, 45, 48, 73, 78, 85, 86, 94, 133, 134, 152; supply and financing of, as affecting quality of service by, 117; U.S. medical care tilted toward, 45, 86–87, 167. *See also specific specialties*

spinal abnormalities, 43–45

spinal-fusion surgery, 19

SSRIs (serotonin uptake inhibitors), 42, 77, 78, 140–41, 171, 198n31

Stamm, Stanley, 25

Starr, Paul, 147

State Children's Health Insurance Program (SCHIP), 37–38, 162, 163, 185

states: health groups' lobbying of, 155; income inequalities between, 58; and managed care, 153; and Medicaid, 12, 30, 68, 79, 103–4, 108, 131, 135–37, 163, 180, 182–85; nurse-patient ratios mandated in some, 187; purchasing of drugs by, from abroad, 171; quality-of-care information in, 33; responsibility of, for mental

States *(continued)*
  illness treatments, 68, 73, 79, 83;
  subsidizing of health care by, 29, 162.
  See also Children's Health Insurance
  Program; *specific states*
statins, 42, 91, 118–19
stent-grafts, 3
Stevens, Rosemary, 15
stress, 40, 56, 58, 72, 143. *See also*
  environment
strokes, 41, 42, 53
Sturm, Heidrun, 131, 132
subspecialties (medical), 87–88
substance abuse (alcohol and/or drug use),
  170; advocates for people suffering from,
  81; clean needles for, 63; costs of
  treatment for, 67; exclusion of treatment
  for, from many insurance plans, 6, 23,
  133, 135; as health risk, 7, 8, 13, 36, 56;
  and mental illness, 77, 79–80; Mormon
  stance on, 65; stigmatization of persons
  with, 50; under treatment for, 116
suicide, 78
Supplemental Security Income (SSI), 183
support groups, 43, 82, 89, 169. *See also*
  disease advocacy groups
Supreme Court (U.S.), 103–4, 147
surgery: amount of, related to number of
  surgeons, 117; back, 19–20; cosmetic,
  130, 135, 139; decision aids for, 177;
  errors in, 21; heart, 33, 52, 87, 125–26,
  155; hip, 31, 116, 122; hospital
  performance information on, 31–32;
  knee, 25, 31, 122; needless and
  ineffective, 19–20, 25; pain perception
  following, 44; untested methods of,
  166–67. *See also* technology (new)
Switzerland, 6

Taiwanese, 61
tattoo removal, 139
taxes: Americans' resistance to higher, 23,
  30, 60, 159, 162, 164, 180; credits in, for
  insurance payments, x, 162; as funding
  drug research, 173; as paying for
  Medicare and Medicaid, 144, 164; as
  paying for mental illness treatments, 68;
  as paying for much of health insurance,
  45; proposed, on Medicare, 182;

  subsidies in, for employer-sponsored
  insurance, 23, 29. *See also* wages vs.
  benefits
teamwork: in chronic care, 8–9, 169–70; in
  dealing with mentally ill, 79–81, 106; in
  elder care, 105–6, 109, 112; quality
  medical care linked to, 14, 21–22, 27, 34,
  88, 95, 113, 129, 168, 170; in UK's
  National Health Service, 122. *See also*
  communication; disease management
  programs; hospitals
technology (new): for back pain, 19–20;
  costs associated with, 23–26, 85, 87, 144;
  creation of demand for, 24, 25–26, 29,
  90, 93, 143–44, 176–77; and longevity,
  51; as no more effective than older,
  cheaper, 19–20, 25, 144; as untested, 17,
  24, 48, 90, 144, 165–66, 176, 177; U.S.
  innovation in, 12, 15, 17, 20, 188. *See
  also* advertising; computerization; drugs;
  medical devices; surgery; treatments
television. *See* media
terrorism, 54
thalidomide (drug), 90, 153
Thomas, William, 111
Thorpe, Kenneth E., 175
thyroid cancer, 25
Ticket to Work and Work Incentives
  Improvement Act (1999), 106, 107
tobacco companies, 155
tobacco use (smoking), 7, 8, 52, 56, 64–65,
  93. *See also* substance abuse
tonsillectomy, 25
tooth capping, 136
Topol, Eric, 2
transplantation services, 21, 137–39, 167,
  206n28
treatments: for body enhancement, 93; large
  number of available, 93; for mental
  illness, 68, 72–77; new surgical, 166–67;
  for non-diseases, 39; patients' concerns
  about withholding of, 5, 17, 30–31,
  35–36, 84, 132, 138–40, 164–65, 177;
  patients' demands for specific, 156, 167,
  176–77; patients' right to seek any,
  73–74; physicians as making decisions
  regarding, 34, 46, 47, 90; potentially
  harmful new, 24–26, 45, 88, 90, 141, 177;
  prior authorization for, 27, 28; side

effects of, 50, 92; unnecessary and/or overused, 5, 6, 11, 19–20, 24–25, 33, 34, 38, 45, 48, 84, 88, 92, 113, 116, 135, 141, 162, 165, 176–77; as untested, 166–67. *See also* drugs (pharmaceutical); surgery; technology (new)

trust, 143–58; as based on familiarity, 34, 125; as easily destroyed, 154, 160; erosion of, in U.S., 3–4, 13–14, 34, 146–48, 159; in FDA, 90–91; lack of, among people with stigmatized conditions, 50; media as undermining social, 35–36, 114, 147, 154, 156, 159, 166; need to build, 34, 35–36, 114, 140, 143–58; in patients' friends and relatives, 34, 85, 125, 146, 149, 150, 177; in patients' personal physicians, 34, 35, 91, 114, 125, 143–46, 148–50, 156, 177, 178; types of, 148–52. *See also* social capital

Tupelo (Mississippi), 111–12

ulcer disease, 116, 199n32
underinsured persons, 23, 182, 190n9
unemployed, 164
uninsured persons: attempts to address problems of, x, 162–64; children among, 37–38; employment status of, 6, 163, 209n4; and hospital finances, 155; increased mortality among, 23, 162, 190n8; number of, in the U.S., ix, 6, 20, 23, 133, 179, 188; as unable to afford insurance, 6, 132, 133, 141, 182

United Healthcare, 15
United Kingdom (UK): evidence-based medicine in, 32–33, 96–97, 165; inequalities in, 60; National Health Service in, 33, 86, 96–97, 120–22, 124, 126, 134–35, 168, 176; polypills recommended in, 42, 53; primary care physicians in, 98; Whitehall studies in, 57, 58

United States: changing smoking attitudes in, 64–65; cost of health care in, as percent of gross national product, 23, 29, 139; health care quality in, ix–x, 6, 20, 115, 141, 188; health spending in, 6; impact of values of, on health care system, 1, 5, 15, 17, 22, 23, 30, 60, 159,

162, 164, 180; increasing poverty in, 185; lack of universal insurance in, 6, 15, 22, 27–28, 38, 161, 188; number of uninsured persons in, ix, 6, 20, 23, 133, 179, 188; per-person health care costs in, 20. *See also* government (U.S.); health care system (U.S.); inequality; prison system; states; taxes

U.S. Advisory Committee on Vital and Health Statistics, 108
U.S. Preventive Services Task Force, 93
University of Minnesota, 111
University of Washington Medical School, 137–38
urologists, 26

VA. *See* Veterans Affairs Department
Vermont, 117
Veterans Affairs Department (VA), 37, 120; drug-price bargaining by, 12, 173; medical care program of, 95, 98, 118, 156
Viagra (drug), 82, 130–32, 139
Vietnam War, 147, 155
violence, 51, 53, 58, 80, 81. *See also* guns
Vioxx (drug), 1–3, 91, 153, 171–72
Vista (health record software), 98
Voluntary Chronic Care Improvement Program, 123

wages vs. benefits, 30, 141, 162. *See also* income
Wagner, Edward, 169
Wales, 51, 53. *See also* United Kingdom
Wal-Mart, 163
war (as health issue), 13. *See also specific wars*
waste. *See* treatments: unnecessary and/or overused
Welch, H. Gilbert, 25
Wells, Kenneth B., 198n29
Wellspring Alliance (Wisconsin), 112
Wennberg, John, 117
White, Kerr, 44
Whitehall studies (UK), 57, 58
Wilensky, Gail, 179–80
Wilkinson, Richard, 59
Williams, T. Franklin, 44
Winakur, Jerald, 100
Wisconsin, 31–32, 112

women: as caregivers for the elderly, 102,
    104, 106; education of, as health issue,
    13, 65; homicide risk for, 51; hormone
    replacement therapy for, 26; as
    physicians, 168, 186; treatments plans
    for, 118–19
Women's Health Study, 119
Woolhandler, Steffie, 175
World Health Organization, 13

About the Author

David Mechanic is the Director of the Institute for Health, Health Care Policy, and Aging Research and the René Dubos University Professor of Behavioral Sciences at Rutgers, the State University of New Jersey. He has been elected to the National Academy of Sciences, the American Academy of Arts and Sciences, and the Institute of Medicine. He is the recipient of the Baxter Prize awarded by the Baxter Allegiance Foundation and the Association of University Programs in Health Administration and the Distinguished Investigator Award from AcademyHealth. He has also received major awards for his work from a range of organizations such as the American Public Health Association, the American Psychiatric Association, and the American Sociological Association. A former Robert Wood Johnson Foundation Investigator in Health Policy Research, he has been National Director of the program since 2000.